The Jewels
of
Nizam

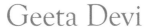

Recipes from the Khansamas of Hyderabad

❀

Geeta Devi

RUPA

Published by
Rupa Publications India Pvt. Ltd 2013
7/16, Ansari Road, Daryaganj
New Delhi 110002

Sales centres:
Allahabad Bengaluru Chennai
Hyderabad Jaipur Kathmandu
Kolkata Mumbai

Copyright © Geeta Devi 2013

Photographs by Sandip Solleti and Ramesh Banala.

ISBN: 978-81-291-2436-4

10 9 8 7 6 5 4 3 2 1

The moral right of the author has been asserted.

Printed at Replika Press Pvt. Ltd., India

Contents

Foreword

The overwhelming demand for her first book, *Dastarkhan-e-Moghlai: 101 Easy to Cook Hyderabadi Recipes*, was so compelling that Smt. Geeta Devi decided to follow it up with *The Jewels of Nizam: Recipes from the Khansamas of Hyderabad*, in which she goes into the past and picks out recipes of the hoary Deccani culture that speak of the richness of its culinary arts. A feature of the recipes is that most of these are little known or forgotten and will be of interest to those fond of Hyderabadi cuisine. They form an enthralling admixture of the past and the present and, in their wholesomeness, will delight those wishing to revive flavours of the past that have been lost in time.

Smt. Geeta Devi has been associated with the Golkonda Hotel, Hyderabad, as a food consultant, and was instrumental in relaunching the Hyderabadi specialty restaurant, Jewel of Nizam. Her recipes are well received by the restaurant clientele and have made the restaurant more popular.

I wish the book every success and hope that Smt. Geeta Devi writes more such volumes that help bring out the latent expertise of the culinary enthusiast.

N. Suresh Reddy
Managing Director
Golkonda Resorts and Spa
Masab Tank
Hyderabad

Introduction

The cuisine of Hyderabad has been refined through centuries, evolving to its current stage owing to both native as well as foreign influences. It was in the medieval era that the foundation of the cuisine was laid—today's Hyderabadi cuisine has a legacy of almost 400 years.

The food that Hyderabad is renowned for today displays a rare yet harmonious blend of Islamic cooking styles and ingredients (Arabic, Mughlai, Turkish and Irani) and indigenous variations from traditional south Indian recipes. It is this spectacular confluence of the foreign and the local that grants to Hyderabadi food its distinctive and unique flavour, and confers—rightly—on it the prestige of being the most exotic cuisine of the Deccan.

My first book, *Dastarkhan-e-Moghlai*, was inspired by my desire to present to food lovers simple delicacies from Hyderabad—recipes that are used every day in Hyderabadi homes to serve up easy-to-prepare yet exquisite dishes. I included in that volume dishes that are popular with one and all, whether from Hyderabad or not, and easy to prepare. It was the success of that book which prompted me to try my hand at reviving some lesser known recipes that originate from the stable of the royal khansamas—richer foods from the courtly tradition of the Nizams.

This book is an attempt to showcase the splendour of Hyderabadi fine dining—the diversity of the cuisine as well as its mouth-watering deliciousness. As you go through the following pages, I hope you will come to agree with me that the food of Hyderabad is indeed the true 'Jewels of Nizam'.

Gazak

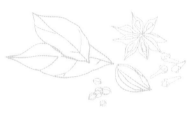

These are appetizers, and this section comprises a selection of recipes for vegetarian and non-vegetarian starters. Traditionally, gazak is served before the main meal and is usually accompanied by a welcome drink. The purpose of gazak is two-fold: while it helps sustain guests before the meal proper is served, it also serves to whet their appetites, with a tantalizing taste of the gastronomical feast that is to follow.

Lamb Cutlets

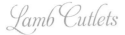

(Patties of minced lamb/chicken/turkey meat)
(6 TO 8 SERVINGS)

Preparation time	20 minutes
Cooking time	20 minutes

INGREDIENTS

Minced meat	500 grams
Tomato	100 grams, cut into small pieces
Black pepper powder	1/2 tsp
Ginger-garlic paste	1 tbsp
Soya sauce	1 tbsp
Worcester sauce	1 tbsp
Maida	as required
Chilli powder	1/2 tsp
Vinegar	1/2 cup (100 ml)
Onion	1, cut into small pieces
Fresh coriander leaves	1/2 cup
Green chillies	3 to 4, cut into small pieces
Bread crumbs	600 grams
Eggs	2
Oil	for frying
Salt	to taste

METHOD

Cook the minced meat with tomatoes, ginger-garlic paste, chilli powder, pepper powder, vinegar, onion, soya sauce, Worcester sauce, fresh coriander leaves, green chillies and salt along with one cup of water, until little water is left in the minced meat. Lower the heat and then add maida, little by little, till the mixture becomes thick. Cool and add two raw eggs and mix well.

Now, make ten to twelve balls out of the minced meat, flatten and roll each ball on the bread crumbs and deep fry. Repeat the process for the remaining mixture.

Serve hot with potato chips.

Gosht ke Lollipop

(Marinated lamb meatballs on sticks)
(4 TO 6 SERVINGS)

Preparation time	10 minutes
Cooking time	40 minutes

INGREDIENTS

Boneless lamb meat (thigh portion)	500 grams, cut into small pieces
Ginger-garlic paste	1 tsp
Chilli powder	1/2 tsp
Turmeric powder	1/2 tsp
Garam masala powder	1/2 tsp
Lemon juice	2 tsp
Oil	for frying
Curd	1 to 2 tsp
Salt	to taste
Narrow wooden sticks	6 to 8 inches long

METHOD

Mix all the ingredients except the curd and oil with the meat pieces and cook in a thick-bottomed vessel with a little water, till the meat becomes tender and the mixture is almost dry. Grind the mixture in a food processor/mixer-grinder till soft. If the mixture is too dry and difficult to grind, add some curd. Make into lemon-sized balls and pierce each one with a stick. Deep fry till golden brown.

Serve hot with mint chutney, tomato ketchup and onion rings.

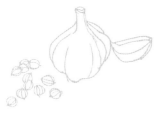

Gosht ka Chudwa

(Fried shredded lamb meat)
(4 TO 6 SERVINGS)

This delicious snack evolved mainly as a way to preserve the abundant quantity of meat available after the sacrifice of goats on certain occasions and festivals.

Preparation time	10 minutes
Cooking time	40 minutes

INGREDIENTS

Boneless lamb meat (thigh portion)	1 kg, cubed
Ginger-garlic paste	1 tbsp
Chilli powder	1 tbsp
Turmeric powder	1/4 tsp
Oil	for frying
Salt	to taste

FOR GARNISHING

Jeera powder
Aamchur powder
Salt
Chilli powder

METHOD

Put the meat pieces, ginger-garlic paste, chilli powder, turmeric powder, salt and two to three cups of water in a pressure cooker. Cook until the meat becomes tender and no water is left in the cooker.

Now shred the meat pieces by hand. Heat oil in a pan and fry these shredded pieces. Place the fried mixture on a paper napkin, so that excess oil is soaked.

Garnish with jeera, aamchur powder and salt. If kept in an airtight jar after cooling, the meat can be stored for eight to ten days.

Patthar ka Gosht

(Lamb meat cooked on stone)
(4 TO 6 SERVINGS)

Mughal royalty, known to be connoisseurs of food, appreciated new dishes and taste. The art of cooking meat by marinating it in a blend of rich spices and grilling it on a hot stone was developed to titillate the taste buds and add a new dimension to the traditional menu. This form of cooking is followed even today.

Preparation time	30 minutes
Cooking time	30 minutes

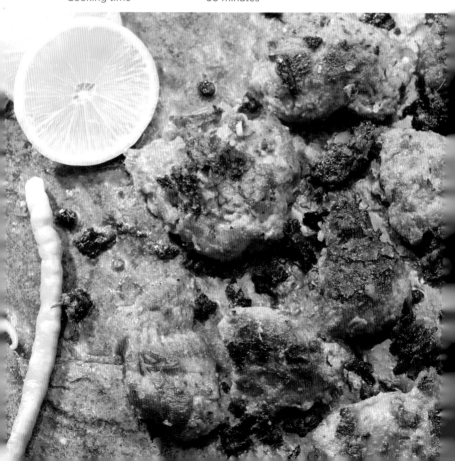

INGREDIENTS

Boneless lamb meat	1 kg cut into medium-sized pieces and flattened
Curd (hung)	1 cup
Garam masala powder	1 tsp
Elaichi powder	1/2 tsp
Green chillies	10-15, grounded into a paste with a bit of salt
Peel of raw papaya	1 tbsp peeled skin paste, for softening meat pieces
Ghee	as required
Salt	to taste

FOR GARNISHING

Onion rings

Lemon wedges

METHOD

Put the meat pieces in a bowl. Mix the curd, green chilli paste, garam masala, elaichi powder, papaya skin paste and salt together and marinate for one-and-a-half to two hours.

Take a seasoned granite stone, about two to two-and-a-half feet long and four to six inches thick. Heat the stone by putting live charcoal below it. Place the pieces of meat on the hot stone and sprinkle some ghee on each side of the meat pieces. Keep turning the pieces until they become crisp and brown.

Serve hot, with onion rings and lemon wedges.

Thatti ka Gosht

(Flattened marinated meat with green chilli paste and spices on a
Hyderabadi style grill)
(6 SERVINGS)

Preparation time	40 minutes
Cooking time	30 minutes

INGREDIENTS

Boneless lamb meat	1 kg, cut into 3 inch pieces and flattened
Dalda ghee	as required
Garam masala powder	1 tsp
Salt	to taste
Green chillies	10 to 15
Coriander leaves	2 tbsp
Mint leaves	2 tbsp

FOR GARNISHING

Onion rings
Lemon wedges

METHOD

Grind to paste, green chillies, coriander leaves and mint leaves, adding
a little salt to the mixture.

Marinate the meat with masala paste, garam masala powder and
salt for two to three hours.

Put the meat pieces in-between the Hyderabadi type grill and cook
on live charcoal, turning frequently while applying ghee with a brush on
the meat pieces, until they become crisp and brown.

Serve hot with onion rings and lemon wedges.

Note: Hyderabadi grill: A rectangular/square grill made of iron rods fixed on one side,
with a clamp to hold the marinated meat pieces in between.

Bheje ke Cutlet

(Lamb brain stuffed in potato)
(4 TO 6 SERVINGS)

Preparation time	10 minutes
Cooking time	20 minutes

INGREDIENTS

Potatoes	500 grams, boiled and peeled
Vinegar	1 tbsp
Black pepper	1/2 tsp
Roasted chana dal (putane ki dal)	50 grams, ground to a powder
Oil	for deep frying
Salt	to taste

FOR STUFFING

Bheja (from lamb)	4, cleaned
Onion	1, cut into small pieces
Black pepper	1/2 tsp
Vinegar	1 tbsp
Oil	2 tbsp
Salt	to taste

METHOD

Mash the potatoes and mix them with vinegar, black pepper, ground chana dal powder and salt. Keep aside.

To make the stuffing, take a pan, add oil and fry the onions. When the onions become translucent, add the bheja. Lower the heat and fry, stirring continuously, till the mixture becomes golden brown. Add the black pepper powder, vinegar and salt.

To make the cutlets, divide the mashed potato mixture into twelve parts. Flatten each portion on the palm and stuff with one to two tablespoons of the cooked bheja mixture, close and flatten the same. Deep fry until the cutlet is golden brown.

Serve hot with mint chutney or tomato ketchup.

Bharwa Murgh Leg

(Stuffed chicken drumsticks)
(4 TO 6 SERVINGS)

Preparation time	10 minutes
Cooking time	20 minutes

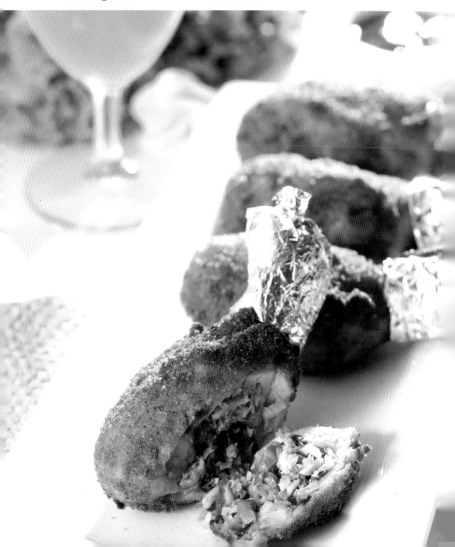

INGREDIENTS

Chicken drumsticks	6 to 8
Minced chicken	150 grams
Onions	1, finely sliced
Ginger-garlic paste	2 tbsp
Chilli powder	1/2 tsp
Green chillies	1 to 2, cut into small pieces
Coriander leaves	2 tbsp, finely chopped
Lemon juice	1 tbsp
Cornstarch	as required
Bread crumbs	as required
Oil	for deep frying
Salt	to taste
Onion	1, cut into rings (for garnishing)

METHOD

Marinate the drumsticks in ginger-garlic paste and salt and keep aside for two hours.

To make the stuffing, place the minced meat in a pan and add chilli powder, salt, green chillies and coriander leaves. Cook till the meat is done and becomes dry. Add lemon juice.

Fill the folds (pockets) of the drumsticks with the stuffing. Mix water with the cornstarch. Dip each stuffed drumstick in the cornstarch and then roll it in bread crumbs. Deep fry till golden brown.

Serve hot with onion rings and pudina chutney.

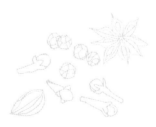

Machli Begum Bahaar

(Fish with pepper and vinegar)
(4 TO 6 SERVINGS)

Preparation time	20 minutes
Cooking time	10 minutes

INGREDIENTS

Fish (fresh water)	1 kg, deboned and cut into 2 inch pieces
Vinegar	2 tbsp
Black pepper powder	1 tsp
Ginger-garlic paste	1 tbsp
Eggs	2, beaten
Oil	for frying
Salt	to taste
Bread crumbs	as required

METHOD

Marinate the fish with ginger-garlic paste, pepper powder, vinegar and salt and keep it aside for one hour.

Dip each piece of marinated fish in the beaten egg, roll it on bread crumbs and deep fry until golden brown.

Serve hot with potato chips.

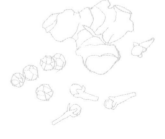

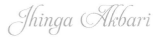

Jhinga Akbari

(Fried spicy prawns)
(4 TO 6 SERVINGS)

Preparation time	30 minutes
Cooking time	15 minutes

INGREDIENTS

Prawns	1 kg, medium-size, shelled and deveined
Ginger-garlic paste	1 tbsp
Green chilli	15 to 20, finely chopped
Fresh coriander leaves	1/2 cup
Chilli powder	1 tsp
Cornflour	1 tbsp
Maida	1 tbsp
Lemon juice	2 tbsp
Oil	for frying
Salt	to taste

METHOD

Take prawns in a vessel. Mix ginger-garlic paste, chilli powder, cornflour, maida, coriander leaves, green chillies, lemon juice and salt with the prawns, and keep aside for one to one-and-a-half hours for marination.

Heat oil in a kadai. Deep fry the prawns, two or three pieces at a time, until they attain a golden brown colour.

Serve hot with mint chutney or tomato sauce.

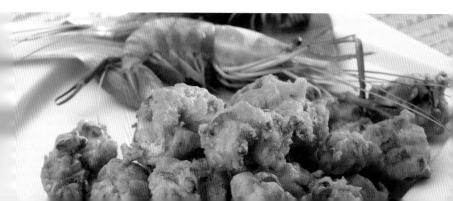

Paneer Golkonda

(Paneer marinated with fresh herbs and spices, and finished in clay oven/tandoor)
(4 TO 6 SERVINGS)

Preparation time	30 minutes
Cooking time	15 minutes

INGREDIENTS

Paneer	500 grams, cut into 2 inch cubes
Green chilli paste	1 tsp (6 to 8 chillies ground to paste)
Ginger-garlic paste	1 tsp
Lemon juice	1 tsp
Garam masala powder	1 tsp
Hung curd	1/2 cup
Fresh coriander leaves	1/2 cup
Salt	to taste
Cream	for garnishing
Butter	for brushing on top

METHOD

Marinate the paneer cubes in green chilli paste, ginger-garlic paste, lemon juice, garam masala powder, fresh coriander leaves, hung curd and salt. Put the marinated paneer pieces on skewers and cook in a clay oven.

Brush with butter and serve with fresh cream.

Fried Baby Corn
(4 TO 6 SERVINGS)

Preparation time	15 minutes
Cooking time	10 minutes

INGREDIENTS

Baby Corn	10 to 15, cut length-wise into half
Oil	for frying
Cornflour	4 tbsp
Maida	4 tbsp
Oil	1 tbsp
Pepper powder	1/2 tsp
Chilli powder	1/2 tsp
Salt	to taste

METHOD

Mix the cornflour, maida, oil, pepper powder, chilli powder and salt together to form a smooth batter. Heat oil in a kadai. Dip each piece of baby corn into the batter and deep fry until golden brown and crisp.

Garnish with chaat masala and serve hot.

Soya Shikampoor

(Soya preparation with masalas)
(4 SERVINGS)

Preparation time	30 minutes
Cooking time	10 minutes

INGREDIENTS

Soya granules	250 grams, soaked overnight
Green chillies	2 to 3, cut into small pieces
Fresh chopped coriander	2 tbsp
Mint leaves	1 tbsp, chopped
Chilli Powder	1 tbsp
Turmeric powder	1/4 tsp
Lemon juice	1 tsp
Roasted Bengal gram	4 tbsp, powdered
Oil	for frying
Salt	to taste

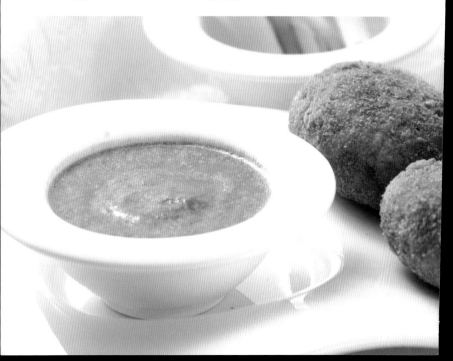

FOR THE STUFFING

Hung curd	1/2 cup
Onion	1, cut into small pieces
Green chillies	1, cut into small pieces
Fresh coriander	1 tbsp

METHOD

Mix all the ingredients for the stuffing together. Now take a pan and cook the drained soya granules, chilli powder, turmeric powder, green chillies, salt, coriander and mint leaves till the water evaporates. Cool and grind into a fine paste. Then add powdered Bengal gram (putane ki dal) and lemon juice and mix well. Take a portion and flatten it on the palm. Add half a teaspoon of the stuffing to it, cover from all sides and flatten it. Deep fry, garnish with chat masala and serve hot with mint chutney.

Note: In case they break, dip the shikampoor in cornflour paste before deep frying.

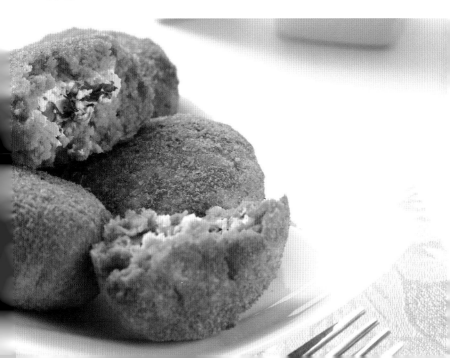

Aamras ke Kofte (Seasonal)

(Minced meatballs cooked with ripe mango pulp)
(4 TO 6 SERVINGS)

This dish is a combination of meatballs and mango pulp. The blend of seasonal mango and mutton cooked on slow flame speaks of the ingenuity of the khansamas, the cooks of the Mughal royalty.

Preparation time	30 minutes
Cooking time	20 minutes

INGREDIENTS

Minced meat (lamb/ chicken)	300 grams, washed and drained
Onion	2, finely chopped
Ginger-garlic paste	1 tbsp
Chilli powder	1 1/2 tbsp
Roasted Bengal gram (putane ki dal)	2 tbsp
Shah jeera	1 tsp
Turmeric powder	1/4 tsp
Oil	1/2 cup
Mango pulp	1/2 cup
Salt	to taste

FOR GARNISHING

Fresh coriander leaves
Mango pieces

METHOD

To make the koftas, in a bowl, mix minced meat, half a tablespoon of chilli powder, Shah jeera, salt and powdered putane ki dal and grind together. Make lemon-sized balls out of the thick mixture and keep aside.

In another vessel, heat oil and fry onions till golden brown. Lower the heat and add ginger-garlic paste, the remaining chilli powder, turmeric powder and salt. Fry together while adding a little water till the oil floats on top. Then add four to five cups of water. When the water boils, add the koftas and cook until the gravy thickens slightly and oil floats on top. Cool a little and then add the mango pulp.

Garnish with coriander and mango pieces and serve hot with chapatis.

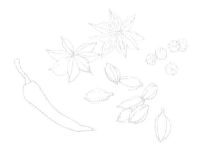

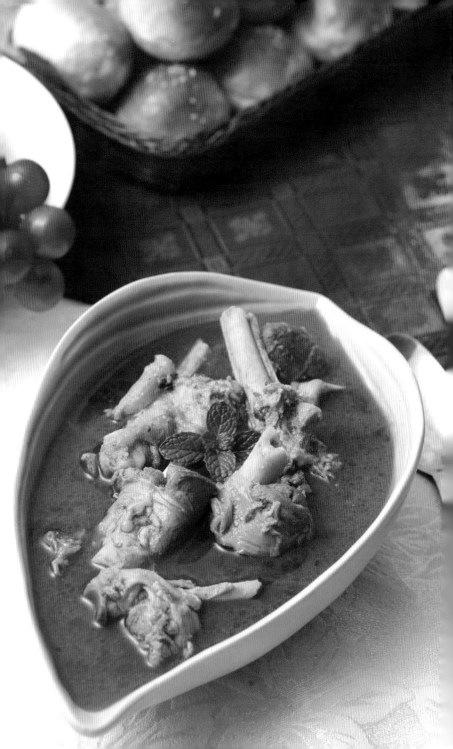

Nalli Boti ka Salan

(Curry of meat with lamb bone marrow)
(4 TO 6 SERVINGS)

Preparation time	10 minutes
Cooking time	30 minutes

INGREDIENTS

Meat with long bone marrow	500 grams, cut so that each piece has bone marrow
Onion	1, finely chopped
Curd	1/2 cup, beaten
Ginger-garlic paste	1 tbsp
Chilli powder	1 tsp
Turmeric powder	1/4 tsp
Khus khus	1 tbsp
Watermelon seeds	2 tbsp
Coriander leaves	1/2 cup
Oil	1/2 cup
Salt	to taste

METHOD

Dry roast and grind to paste, khus khus, watermelon seeds, coriander leaves, oil and salt. Heat oil in a pressure cooker and fry the onions till golden brown. Lower the heat and add ginger-garlic paste, chilli powder, turmeric powder, salt, the pieces of meat, half of the coriander leaves and the ground paste. Fry, adding a little water, till the oil floats on top and the masalas are properly fried. Add two cups of water and pressure cook till the meat is done.

Garnish with coriander leaves and serve hot with chapatis or rice.

Achaari Machli

(Fish cooked in pickle style)
(4 TO 6 SERVINGS)

Preparation time	20 minutes
Cooking time	30 minutes

INGREDIENTS

Fish (fresh water)	1 kg, deboned and cut into 2 inch pieces
Onion	2, cut into slices, deep fried and ground into paste
Chilli powder	2 tbsp
Kalonji	1 tsp
Jeera and rai	1 tsp
Oil	1 cup
Lemon juice	1/2 cup
Salt	to taste

METHOD

In a non-stick pan, heat 3 tbsp of oil, sauté the fish pieces and keep aside.

In another vessel, pour the remaining oil. Add jeera, rai and kalonji and heat on a flame. When they crackle, add onion paste, chilli powder and salt, stirring continuously till the oil floats.

Lower the heat, add the fish pieces and stir slowly, without breaking the pieces. Cook till the fish is done.

Add lemon juice and serve hot with rice or chapatis.

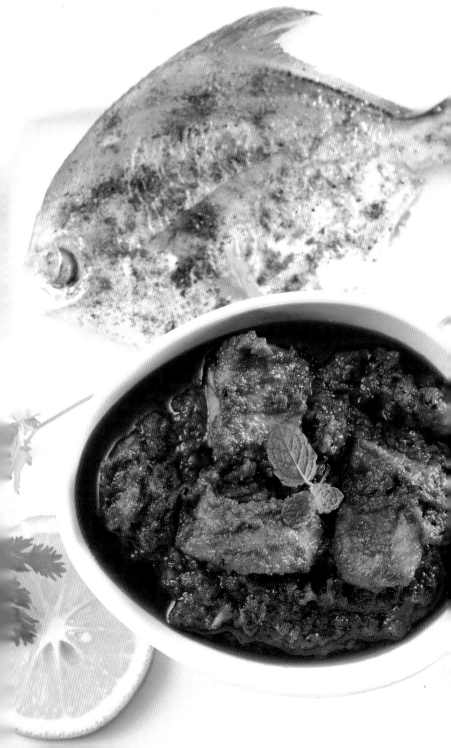

Nargisi Kebab ka Korma

(Lamb meat and boiled egg curry)
(4 TO 6 SERVINGS)

Preparation time	30 minutes
Cooking time	30 minutes

INGREDIENTS

Eggs	6, boiled and peeled
Boneless lamb meat	200 grams, pressure cooked with a little salt, chilli powder, ginger-garlic paste and water till tender, then ground to a thick fine paste
Onion	1, finely chopped
Ginger-garlic paste	1 tbsp
Chilli powder	1 tsp
Turmeric powder	1/4 tsp
Curd	1/2 cup, beaten
Roasted Bengal gram (putane ki dal)	1 tbsp, powdered
Oil	for frying and cooking
Salt	to taste
Khus khus	1 tbsp
Watermelon seeds	1 tbsp

METHOD

To make the kebabs, add the powdered Bengal gram powder to the meat paste. Mix thoroughly and make six balls out of the mixture. Cover each boiled egg with one portion of the meat mixture. Deep fry till golden brown and keep aside.

Dry roast the khus khus and watermelon seeds and grind them to paste.

To make the gravy, heat oil in a pan and fry onions till golden brown. Lower the heat and add ginger-garlic paste, chilli powder, turmeric powder, salt and the ground paste. Fry, adding a little water, until the oil floats on top. Then add the beaten curd. Continue to fry the mixture. After the masala is cooked, add one cup of water. Continue to cook until the gravy is half thickened.

To serve, cut the kebabs into two halves. Place them in a bowl and pour the gravy over it. Garnish with coriander and serve hot with chapatis or rice.

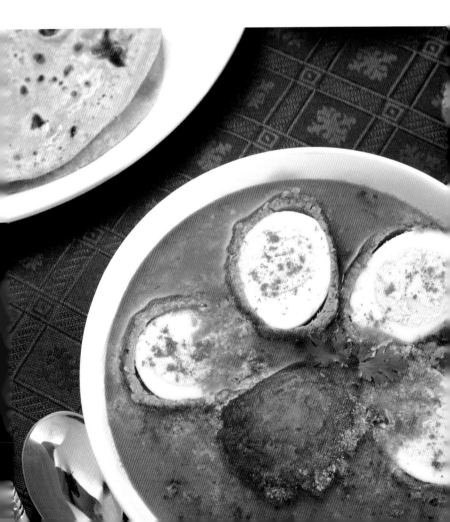

Vegetarian Fish

(Fried yam)
(4 TO 6 SERVINGS)

Preparation time	30 minutes
Cooking time	10 minutes

INGREDIENTS

Yam (jimikand)	1 kg, boiled, peeled and cut into 3 inch slices
Vinegar	2 tbsp
Pepper powder	1 tsp
Oil	for frying
Bread crumbs	as required
Cornflour	2 to 3 tbsp
Salt	to taste

METHOD

Soak the yam pieces in a mixture of vinegar, pepper and salt for ten to fifteen minutes. Make a thick paste of cornflour, dip a piece in the paste, roll it over the bread crumbs and deep fry. Repeat for all the other pieces.

Sprinkle chaat masala and serve hot.

Magzeyti Dulme

(Lamb meat preparation with dry fruits)
(4 TO 6 SERVINGS)

Mughlai cuisine is known for its rich taste and exotic flavours. In this preparation, a blend of nuts and spices are rolled in mutton pieces and cooked in thick gravy till the meat gets tender. It speaks of the great appreciation the royalty had for variety, flavour and spices.

Preparation Time	30 minutes
Cooking Time	20 minutes

INGREDIENTS

Boneless lamb meat	400 grams, cut into slices
Ginger-garlic paste	1 tbsp
Black pepper powder	1 Tsp
Turmeric powder	1/4 tsp
Oil	1 cup
Mixed dry fruits (pista, badaam, kaju)	1/2 cup, finely chopped with a little salt
White vinegar	2 tbsp
Salt	to taste
Thread	for tying the dulme

METHOD

Flatten each piece of meat and place half a teaspoon of chopped dry fruit in the centre. Fold the meat pieces from the side and tie with the thread. Do the same with all the meat pieces and keep aside.

Put oil in the pressure cooker. Fry onions till golden brown. Lower the heat and add ginger-garlic paste, pepper powder, turmeric powder and salt. Keep adding small amounts of water till the oil floats on top. Then add vinegar and fry a little more. Add the dulme along with three cups of water. Cook until the meat is done. Serve hot with chapatis.

Note: If more water is left after cooking, cook further to reduce the water till gravy thickens.

Main Course

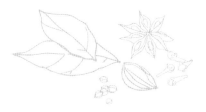

This section is again divided into two parts, non-vegetarian and vegetarian. The non-vegetarian recipes comprise preparations of succulent and tender flesh of lamb, chicken or fish, cooked with flavourful mixes of spices. The vegetarian items too will delight gourmands, with uncommon and innovative recipes for vegetables such as capsicum, beet and tomato, as well as paneer, soya and besan.

Chirongi ka Dalcha

(Chirongi lamb meat curry)
(4 TO 6 SERVINGS)

This delicacy, with its subtle flavours of nuts combined with meat, was popular during the Nizam's reign. It was believed that the dal (lintel), generally used to make dalcha, causes joint pains and, hence, chirongi (piyal nut), which is the same shape as dal, was used as a substitute in its place. It is what gives the dish its rich taste.

Preparation time	10 minutes
Cooking time	30 minutes

INGREDIENTS

Boneless lamb meat	250 grams, cut into cubes
Onion	1, cut into thin slices
Ginger-garlic paste	1 tbsp
Chilli powder	1 tsp
Turmeric powder	1/4 tsp
Oil	1/2 cup
Chirongi seeds	100 grams, soaked overnight and dehusked
Curd	1/2 cup, beaten
Fresh coriander leaves	2 tbsp
Salt	to taste

METHOD

Heat oil in a pressure cooker and fry onions till golden brown. Lower the heat and add ginger-garlic paste. Keep adding small amounts of water. Now add chilli powder, turmeric powder and salt, along with the meat pieces. Stir until the oil floats on top. Then add curd and fry till the raw smell goes. Add the chirongi and two cups of water. Cook until the meat is done.

Garnish with coriander and serve hot with rice or chapatis.

Double Beans aur Keema

(Minced meat with broad beans) (Lamb/chicken/turkey)
(4 TO 6 SERVINGS)

Preparation time	15 minutes
Cooking time	30 minutes

INGREDIENTS

Meat	250 grams, minced
Double beans	200 grams, fresh or dried, soaked in water overnight and boiled
Onion	1, finely sliced
Ginger-garlic paste	1 tbsp
Turmeric powder	1/2 tsp
Chilli powder	1 tsp
Oil	1/2 cup
Chopped coriander leaves	2 tbsp
Salt	to taste

METHOD

Heat oil in a pan, add onions and fry till golden brown. Add ginger-garlic paste, lower the heat and stir, sprinkling a little water. Add chilli powder, turmeric powder, salt and the minced meat. Continue to stir for two to three minutes and then add the double beans and half of the coriander leaves, with half a cup of water. Cook until the water evaporates and the beans are done.

Garnish with coriander leaves and serve hot with chapatis or rice.

Note: In case of fresh broad beans, use only the seeds for the recipe.

Machli ka Pulusu
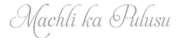

(Spicy fish curry)
(4 TO 6 SERVINGS)

Preparation time	20 minutes
Cooking time	20 minutes

INGREDIENTS

Fish (preferably a hard variety like rohu)	1 kg, cleaned and cut into medium slices and sautéed
Onion	2, finely sliced
Tamarind pulp	1/2 cup
Ginger-garlic paste	1 tbsp
Chilli powder	1 tbsp
Turmeric powder	1/2 tsp
Dhania powder	1 tsp
Roasted Bengal gram (putane ki dal)	1 tsp, powdered
Methi powder	1/4 tsp
Jeera powder	1 tsp
Green chillies	2 to 3, slit into halves
Curry leaves	4 to 6
Jeera and rai	1 tsp
Oil	1/2 cup
Salt	to taste

METHOD

Heat oil in a pan and add the jeera, rai, curry leaves and onions. Fry till golden brown and then add the ginger-garlic paste. Lower the heat and add chilli powder, turmeric powder, salt, jeera powder, dhania powder, methi powder, powdered Bengal gram (putane ki dal) and fry a little. Then add tamarind pulp, green chillies and fry for two to three minutes. Add two cups of water and cook till the mixture reduces to half and becomes thick. Add the fish pieces and simmer for two to three minutes.

Serve hot with rice.

Milwa Bhaji ka Kalia

(Green leafy vegetables cooked with meat)
(4 TO 6 SERVINGS)

Preparation time	20 minutes
Cooking time	30 minutes

INGREDIENTS

Spinach	2 bunches
Amarant (Maat ki bhaji)	2 bunches
Kulfe ke bhaji	2 bunches
Chukka ki bhaji	2 bunches
Methi leaves	2 bunches
(fenugreek leaves)	
Green chillies	2, slit into halves
Ambada leaves	1 cup
(roselle leaves)	
Boneless lamb meat	200 grams, cut into small pieces
Onion	1, finely sliced
Ginger-garlic paste	1 tbsp
Tomato	1, cut into small pieces
Chilli powder	1 tbsp
Turmeric powder	1/2 tsp
Oil	1/2 cup
Salt	to taste

METHOD

Wash the greens and cut them into small pieces. Heat oil in a pressure cooker and fry the onions till golden brown. Add ginger-garlic paste, lower the heat and then add chilli powder, turmeric powder, salt, meat pieces, tomato and green chillies and fry for two to three minutes. Add all the washed and cut greens together with the ambada leaves. Pressure cook till the meat is done. If required, add a little water. Cook till the oil floats on the top.

Serve hot with rice.

Chakna

(Mixed spare-parts lamb curry)
(4 TO 6 SERVINGS)

It is a ritual to sacrifice goats on certain festivals. The lean meat is used in the preparation of curries while the visceral parts are cooked in a gravy of gram flour, pure ghee and spices to make an ideal dish to serve with rotis.

Preparation time	20 minutes
Cooking time	30 minutes

INGREDIENTS

Lamb chops	200 grams, boiled
Kidneys (lamb)	100 grams, cut into 2 halves
Liver (lamb)	100 grams, cut into 2 inch pieces
Tongue (lamb)	2, boiled and peeled and cut into 2 halves
Boneless Chicken	200 grams, cut into 1 inch pieces
Onion	2, finely sliced
Ginger-garlic paste	1 tbsp
Chilli powder	1 tsp
Turmeric powder	1/2 tsp
Green chillies	2 to 3, cut into small pieces
Coriander leaves	1/2 tbsp, finely chopped
Lemon juice	2 tbsp
Bengal gram flour (besan)	2 tbsp, roasted in 2 tbsp of pure ghee
Curd	1/2 cup, beaten
Oil	1/2 cup
Salt	to taste

METHOD

Heat oil in a pan and fry the onions till golden brown. Remove half of the fried onions and keep aside. Keep the other half of the fried onions in the pan and add the ginger-garlic paste. Fry a little, lower the heat and add chilli powder, turmeric powder, salt and continue frying for two to three minutes. Then add the liver and kidneys. Fry a little and add the beaten curd. Cook till the oil floats on top. Then add the chicken and two cups of water. Cook for a few minutes till the chicken is half done and then add the lamb chops and tongue.

Make a paste out of the gram flour by mixing it with one cup of water and add this mixture to the gravy, stirring continuously so that no lumps are formed. Add lemon juice, mix well and cook till the oil floats on top.

Serve hot after garnishing with fried onions and coriander leaves.

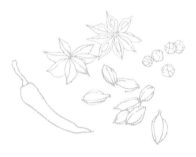

Kadai ke Bheje
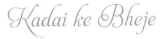

(Lamb brain cooked with masalas)
(4 TO 6 SERVINGS)

Preparation time	10 minutes
Cooking time	20 minutes

INGREDIENTS

Bheja (lamb brain)	4, cleaned and deveined
Onion	6 to 7, finely sliced
Black pepper	1 tbsp
Turmeric powder	1/2 tsp
Vinegar	1 tbsp
Oil	3/4 cup
Salt	to taste

METHOD

Fry onions in a pan till they turn translucent. Lower the heat and add the bheja. Stir occasionally and cook till the onions are golden brown and the bheja is cooked. Add black pepper, turmeric powder and salt. Fry a little and then add vinegar. Stir till the curry becomes dry and the oil floats on top.

Serve hot with puris.

Kulfe ki Bhaji ka Kalia

(Lamb meat curry with kulfe leaves)
(4 TO 6 SERVINGS)

Preparation time	10 minutes
Cooking time	30 minutes

INGREDIENTS

Kulfe ki bhaji	500 grams or 4 to 5 bunches, washed and cut into small pieces
Boneless lamb meat	200 grams, cut into small pieces
Tomato	1, cut into small pieces
Onion	2, finely cut
Ginger-garlic paste	1 tbsp
Chilli powder	1 tbsp
Turmeric powder	1/2 tsp
Aamchur (dried mango)	5 to 6 pieces, soaked in water
or fresh mango	1 slice, chopped
Oil	1/2 cup
Salt	to taste

METHOD

Heat oil in a pan and fry the onions till golden brown. Then add the ginger-garlic paste. Lower the heat and add turmeric powder, chilli powder, aamchur, salt and the meat pieces and cook for one to two minutes. Then add the tomato and bhaji and cover with a lid. Stir for two or three minutes, add a cup of water and cook till the meat is done and the oil floats on top.

Serve hot with rice.

Gajar-Methi ka Salan

(Carrot-fenugreek curry)
(4 TO 6 SERVINGS)

Preparation time	20 minutes
Cooking Time	30 minutes

INGREDIENTS

Gajar (carrot)	500 grams; peel the skin, remove the centre bone and cut into small pieces
Boneless lamb meat	150 grams, cut into small pieces
Fresh methi leaves	1/2 cup
Fresh shelled peas or green chana	1/2 cup
Tomato	1, cut into small pieces
Onion	1, finely cut
Ginger-garlic paste	1 tbsp
Chilli powder	1 tsp
Turmeric powder	1/2 tsp
Oil	1/2 cup
Lemon juice	1 tbsp
Salt	to taste

METHOD

Heat oil in a thick-bottomed pan and fry the onions till golden brown. Add ginger-garlic paste, lower the heat and then add turmeric powder, chilli powder, salt, methi leaves and tomato. Fry for about one or two minutes. Add the meat, fry a little and then add one cup of water. Cover with a lid and cook until the meat is done. Then add the gajar and peas/chana. If necessary, add a little water, cover and cook till the water evaporates and the oil floats on top.

Add lemon juice and serve hot with rice.

Safed Gosht ka Salan

(Lamb meat cooked with curds and green chillies)
(4 TO 6 SERVINGS)

Preparation time	20 minutes
Cooking time	30 minutes

INGREDIENTS

Lamb meat with bones	500 grams, cut into medium-sized pieces
Curd	250 grams, beaten
Green chillies	6 to 8, ground to paste with some salt
Cream	1/2 cup
Oil	1/2 cup
Onion	2, cut into thin slices
Garam masala (whole)	1/2 tsp
Ginger-garlic paste	1 tbsp
Salt	to taste
Coriander leaves	for garnishing
Khus khus	2 tbsp
Watermelon seeds	2 tbsp

METHOD

Dry roast the khus khus and watermelon seeds and grind them to paste.

Heat oil in a pressure cooker. Add the onions and fry till translucent. Add ginger-garlic paste, garam masala and fry a little. Add the meat pieces and salt and fry for two to three minutes. Lower the heat and add the beaten curd, green chilli paste and the dry roasted paste and fry till the oil floats on top. Add two to three cups of water and cook until the meat is done.

Garnish with cream and fresh coriander leaves and serve hot with chapatis.

Turai-Ande ka Salan

(Curry of ridge gourd and egg)
(4 TO 6 SERVINGS)

Preparation time	20 minutes
Cooking time	20 minutes

INGREDIENTS

Turai (ridge gourd)	1 kg, peeled and cut into small pieces
Methi leaves	1 small bunch, approx. 1/2 cup
Eggs	6, boiled and peeled, with cuts made on the outer surface
Onion	1, sliced finely
Tomato	1, finely chopped
Ginger-garlic paste	1 tbsp
Chilli powder	1 tsp
Turmeric powder	1/2 tsp
Oil	1/2 cup
Salt	to taste

METHOD

Heat oil in a heavy-bottomed pan and fry the onions till golden brown. Add ginger-garlic paste and fry, sprinkling a little water. Lower the heat and add chilli powder, turmeric powder, salt, methi leaves and tomato. Fry for two to three minutes and add a little water if required. Add turai, mix well, cover with a lid and cook on a low flame till the turai is soft and done. Then add the boiled eggs.

Serve hot with rice or chapatis.

Zabaan ka Korma

(Lamb tongue curry)
(4 TO 6 SERVINGS)

Preparation time	20 minutes
Cooking time	20 minutes

INGREDIENTS

Zabaan (lamb tongue)	6, boiled, peeled and cut into halves
Onion	2, finely sliced
Ginger-garlic paste	1 tbsp
Chilli powder	1 tsp
Turmeric powder	1/2 tsp
Garam masala (whole)	1 tsp
Curd	250 grams, beaten
Oil	1/2 cup
Fresh coriander leaves	1/2 cup
Salt	to taste
Khus khus	1 tbsp
Watermelon seeds	1 tbsp

METHOD

Dry roast the khus khus and watermelon seeds and grind them to paste.

Heat oil in a deep pan and fry the onions till golden brown. Add ginger-garlic paste and fry, sprinkling a little water. Lower the heat and add chilli powder, turmeric powder, salt and half of the coriander leaves. Fry for a minute, then add the ground paste, garam masala and a little water and continue frying for a few minutes till the oil floats on top. Add the curd and cook for a couple of minutes. Then add one cup of water and cook till the oil floats on top. Finally, add the boiled tongue and the remaining coriander leaves and cook for a minute.

Serve hot with rice after garnishing with coriander leaves.

Chakoli

(Preparation of raw wheat chapatis and meat) (Lamb/chicken)
(4 TO 6 SERVINGS)

This dish is a meal by itself. Prepared to replace the ordeal of making rotis as well as an accompanying dish, the combined taste of wheat flour and meat blended in a gravy of yogurt adds variety to the daily menu.

Preparation time	30 minutes
Cooking time	30 minutes

INGREDIENTS

Wheat flour	200 grams
Boneless meat	200 grams, cut into small pieces
Curd	250 grams, beaten
Onion	1, chopped
Tomato	1, cut into small pieces
Potato	1, cut into 1½ inch cubes
Ginger-garlic paste	1 tbsp
Chilli powder	1/2 tsp
Turmeric powder	1/2 tsp
Coriander leaves	1/2 cup, finely chopped
Oil	1/2 cup
Salt	to taste
Lemon juice	for garnishing

METHOD

To make the chakoli, add salt to the flour and prepare a soft dough with a little water. Make six to eight balls. Roll each ball into flat, round shapes like chapatis and cut into one-inch diamond or square pieces.

To make the gravy, heat oil in a pan, add the onions and fry till golden brown. Add ginger-garlic paste and lower the heat. Sprinkle a little water and stir. Now add the chilli powder, turmeric powder, salt, tomato, potato, half of the coriander leaves and meat pieces. Continue to stir for two or three minutes and then add the curd. Cook for about four minutes. Then add four or five cups of water and cook with the lid on till the meat is done (a pressure cooker can be used for this purpose as well). Open the lid and add the chakoli pieces. Cook on medium flame till the gravy becomes semi-thick. Garnish with coriander leaves and lemon juice.

Note: Allow the gravy to be slightly liquid in consistency as it thickens when it cools. This is a whole meal by itself.

To make it a vegetarian dish, the meat can be substituted with potatoes.

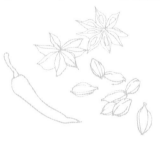

Kofta aur Dahi-ki-Kadi

(Meatballs in curd preparation) (Lamb/chicken/turkey)
(4 TO 6 SERVINGS)

Preparation time	30 minutes
Cooking time	30 minutes

INGREDIENTS

Minced meat	250 grams
Curd	500 grams, beaten
Bengal gram flour	4 to 5 tbsp
Jeera, rai	1 tsp
Ginger	8 to 10, 1/4 inch to 1/2 inch pieces
Curry leaves	10 to 12
Green chillies	2 to 3, slit into halves
Dry red chillies	4 to 5
Chilli powder	1 tsp
Turmeric powder	1/2 tsp
Oil	1/4 cup
Fresh coriander leaves	2 tbsp, finely chopped
Salt	to taste

METHOD

To make the meatballs, mix the minced meat with one tablespoon of gram flour, half a teaspoon of chilli powder and salt. Grind to a fine paste and make lemon-sized balls. Deep fry and keep aside to cool.

To make the kadi, in a bowl, add the curd mixed with the remaining gram flour, salt, chilli and turmeric powder. Mix well and add two to three cups of water.

Heat oil in a deep pan and add jeera, rai, curry leaves and dry red chillies. When the masalas crackle, add the curd mixture. Stir continuously and add the ginger pieces, green chillies and coriander leaves. Cook till the mixture becomes slightly thick. Remove from the flame and add the meatballs.

Serve hot with rice.

Haleem

(Broken wheat and lamb meat preparation)
(6 TO 8 SERVINGS)

This delicious preparation of whole wheat, nuts and mutton, mostly prepared and eaten in the month of Ramadan, is made in pure ghee. Its rich, high satiety value helps offset hunger during the fasting period. The slow cooking brings out the flavours of the mutton and the spices.

Preparation time	40 minutes
Cooking time	60 minutes

INGREDIENTS

Medium wheat rawa	250 grams
Boneless lamb meat	750 grams, cut into small pieces
Curd	250 grams, beaten
Ginger-garlic paste	1 tbsp
Chilli powder	1 tsp
Turmeric powder	1/2 tsp
Onion	2 to 3, cut into thin slices; deep fry half to golden brown and keep the remaining for garnishing
Oil	1/2 cup
Garam masala powder	1 tsp
Pure ghee	150 grams
Milk	200 ml
Lemon juice	1/4 cup
Fresh coriander leaves	2 bunches
Mint leaves	1/2 cup
Green chillies	4 to 6, cut into small pieces
Salt	to taste

METHOD

Soak the wheat rawa overnight and cook with water until soft. In a thick-bottomed pan or pressure cooker, add oil, the remaining half of the fried onions, ginger-garlic paste and stir while adding a little water. Lower the heat, add turmeric powder, chilli powder, garam masala powder, salt and stir. Then add the meat and stir for some time. Add the beaten curd and stir for another two to three minutes. Adding two cups of water, pressure cook until the meat becomes tender.

Grind the cooked wheat and the cooked meat together in a thick-bottomed vessel, mixing them thoroughly. Add the fresh coriander leaves, mint leaves, green chillies, milk and ghee. Mix well till it becomes semi-liquid. Add a little water if required. Cook the mixture on medium flame, stirring continuously till the oil floats on top.

Garnish with fresh coriander leaves, fried onions, fried cashew nuts (optional) and lemon juice. Serve hot.

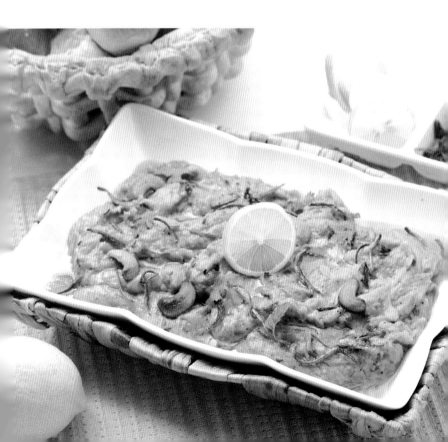

Hari-Mirchi ke Jhinge

(Prawns cooked in green chillies)
(4 TO 6 SERVINGS)

Preparation Time	20 minutes
Cooking Time	20 minutes

INGREDIENTS

Fresh prawns	500 grams, shelled and deveined
Onion	2, finely sliced
Ginger-garlic paste	1 tbsp
Turmeric powder	1/2 tsp
Lemon juice	2 to 4 tbsp
Oil	1/2 cup
Shah jeera	1 tsp
Salt	to taste
Green chillies	8 to 10
Fresh coriander leaves	2 tbsp
Khus khus	2 tbsp
Watermelon seeds	2 tbsp

METHOD

Grind the chillies and coriander leaves to paste. Also dry roast the khus khus and watermelon seeds and grind them to paste.

Fry the onions in oil till golden brown. Add ginger-garlic paste, fry a little and lower the heat. Now add the green chilli paste, ground dry roast paste, turmeric and salt. Fry while adding a little water and then add the prawns. Cook until the prawns are soft and cooked through.

Add lemon juice and serve hot with rice.

Murgh Jalfarezi

(Chicken cooked with ginger and dry whole masala)
(4 TO 6 SERVINGS)

Preparation time	30 minutes
Cooking time	30 minutes

INGREDIENTS

Chicken with bones	750 grams, cut into medium-sized pieces
Fresh ginger	100 grams, cut into thin strips
Pepper (whole)	2 tbsp
Dry red chillies	10 to 12, sticks to be removed
Onion	2, cut into rings
Dhania (whole)	1 tbsp
Oil	3/4 cup
Curd	1/2 cup, beaten
Fresh coriander leaves	1/2 cup
Salt	to taste

METHOD

Heat oil in a heavy-bottomed pan. Add the chicken and cook till it is about three-fourths done. Lower the heat and add ginger, onions, peppercorn, dhania, red chillies, salt and curd. Cook, till the chicken is done, stirring occasionally.

Garnish with cream and fresh coriander leaves and serve hot with chapatis.

Kali-Mirch ke Chops

(Mutton cooked with black pepper) (Lamb)
(4 TO 6 SERVINGS)

Preparation time	10 minutes
Cooking time	30 minutes

INGREDIENTS

Lamb chops	500 grams, flattened
Onion	2, cut into small pieces
Black pepper powder	1 tsp
Turmeric powder	1/2 tsp
Ginger-garlic paste	1 tbsp
Vinegar	1/4 cup
Oil	1/2 cup
Salt	to taste

METHOD

Heat oil in a heavy-bottomed pan and fry the onions till golden brown. Lower the heat, add the ginger-garlic paste and fry for a minute. Now add turmeric powder, pepper powder, salt and lamb chops. Fry for two to three minutes, add vinegar and continue frying for another minute or two. Add two or three cups of water and cook till the chops are done and the oil floats on top.

Serve hot with chapatis after garnishing with potato wedges (optional).

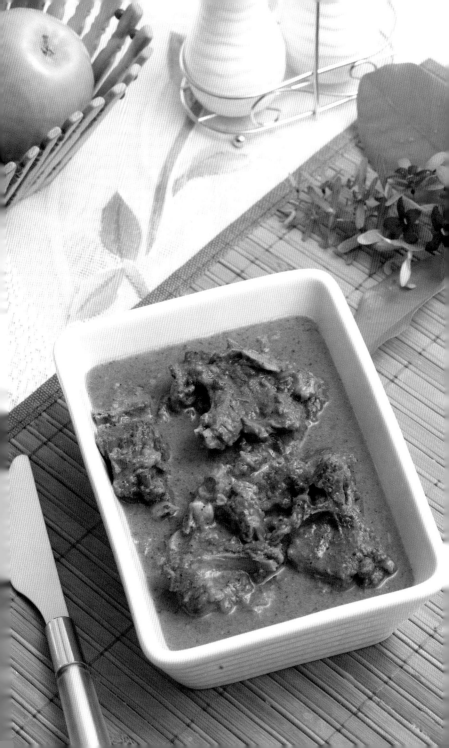

Chippe ka Murgh

(Chicken cooked in an earthen pot)
(4 TO 6 SERVINGS)

Preparation time	10 minutes
Cooking time	20 minutes

INGREDIENTS

Chicken (with or without bones)	750 grams, cut into medium-sized pieces
Ginger-garlic paste	2 tbsp
Chilli powder	1 tsp
Turmeric powder	1/2 tsp
Ghee	4 tbsp
New flat earthen pot, preferably with a lid	1
Salt	to taste

FOR GARNISHING

Onion rings
Lemon wedges
Fresh coriander leaves

METHOD

Take chicken in a bowl. Mix ginger-garlic paste, chilli powder, turmeric powder and salt and marinate for one hour.

Wash the earthen pot and place it on a low flame. Add ghee and the marinated chicken, mixing well. Now cover the pot with the lid and cook, stirring occasionally till the chicken is cooked.

Garnish with onion rings, lemon wedges and coriander leaves and serve the dish in the same pot.

Murgh Kaju ka Korma

(Chicken cooked with cashew paste)
(4 TO 6 SERVINGS)

Preparation time	20 minutes
Cooking time	30 minutes

INGREDIENTS

Chicken with bone	750 grams, cut into medium pieces
Onion	1, finely chopped
Ginger-garlic paste	1 tbsp
Chilli powder	1 tbsp
Turmeric powder	1/4 cup
Oil	1/2 cup
Cashew pieces	100 grams; few pieces to be fried and kept for garnishing, remaining to be ground
Garam masala (whole)	1 tsp
Curd	1/2 cup, beaten
Coriander leaves	for garnishing
Salt	to taste

METHOD

Heat oil in a pan. Add the onions along with the garam masala. When half cooked, add the pieces of chicken. When the water from the chicken dries up, add ginger-garlic paste, turmeric powder, chilli powder and salt. Mix a little water and stir. Add two cups of water and cook till it is about three-fourths done. Then add the cashew paste, stirring continuously on a low heat till the oil floats on top and the chicken is cooked.

Garnish with fried cashew and coriander leaves and serve with rice or chapatis.

Lal Murgh

(Chicken in red chilli paste)
(4 TO 6 SERVINGS)

Preparation time	30 minutes
Cooking time	30 minutes

INGREDIENTS

Chicken with bone	750 grams, cut into medium-sized pieces
Dry red chillies	20 to 25, soaked in water and ground into paste
Onion	1, cut into fine pieces
Ginger-garlic paste	1 tbsp
Turmeric powder	1/4 tsp
Oil	3/4 cup
Lemon juice	2 tbsp
Fresh coriander leaves	for garnishing
Salt	to taste

METHOD

Heat oil in a pan and cook the onions till they are half done. Add the pieces of chicken, stirring continuously till the chicken is almost cooked. Then add the ginger-garlic paste, red chilli paste, turmeric powder and salt. Add a little water and continue to stir till the chicken is fully cooked. If the chicken is not cooked, add a little more water and cook till the oil floats on top. Add lemon juice.

Garnish with coriander leaves and serve hot with chapatis.

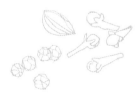

Mahi Murgh ka Salan

(Chicken cooked with bhagara masala)
(4 TO 6 SERVINGS)

This dish adds variety to the non-vegetarian menu and offers flavours and tastes that is appealing to even the most discerning palates.

Preparation time	30 minutes
Cooking time	15 minutes

INGREDIENTS

Boneless chicken	500 grams, cut into medium-sized pieces
Onion	1, cut into thin slices
Ginger-garlic paste	1 tbsp
Chilli powder	1 tsp
Turmeric powder	1/4 tsp
Tamarind pulp	1/2 cup
Curry leaves	8 to 10
Oil	1/2 cup
Jeera and rai	1 tsp (mixed)
Salt	to taste
Peanuts	2 tbsp
Khus khus	1 tbsp
Til (sesame seeds)	1 tbsp
Dry coconut	2 pieces, approx. 2 inches each
Dhania	1 tbsp
Jeera	1 tbsp

METHOD

Dry roast and grind to paste peanuts, khus khus, til, dry coconut dhania and jeera.

Heat oil in a pan and add jeera, rai and curry leaves to it. When they crackle, add the onions and fry till golden brown. Lower the heat; now add ginger-garlic paste, chilli powder, turmeric powder, salt and the ground paste. Fry, adding a little water, till the raw smell goes. Then add the chicken pieces and the tamarind pulp. Continue frying by adding water and cook until the chicken is done and the oil floats on top.

Serve hot with rice.

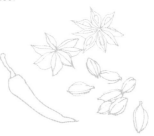

Bharwa Murgh

(Stuffed chicken)
(4 TO 6 SERVINGS)

A delicious dish that was originally served as a snack to the guests of royalty. Chicken is stuffed with boiled eggs, nuts, vegetables, etc., with a marinate of spicy sauce. The chicken is then grilled with a spoonful of ghee till done. The dish reflects the respect and honour the royalty had for its guests.

Preparation time	30 minutes
Cooking time	40 minutes

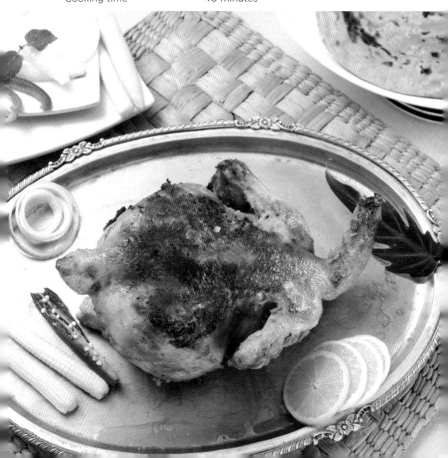

INGREDIENTS

Full chicken without skin	1 kg
Kidneys (lamb)	100 grams, cut into 4 pieces
Liver (lamb)	100 grams, cut into 1 inch pieces
Minced meat (lamb)	50 grams
Eggs	2, boiled
Ginger-garlic paste	2 tbsp
Black pepper	2 tsp
Turmeric powder	1/2 tsp
Vinegar	2 tsp
Soya sauce	1 tsp
Worcester sauce	1 tsp
Onion	2, thinly sliced for frying and garnishing
Oil	2 tbsp
Salt	to taste
Needle and thread	

METHOD

Marinate the chicken for one hour with one tablespoon of ginger-garlic paste and salt and keep aside.

To make the stuffing, heat oil in a pan, add half of the onions to it and fry till golden brown. Lower the heat and add the ginger-garlic paste, pepper, salt and turmeric powder. Fry a little and then add the minced meat, kidneys and liver and one tablespoon of vinegar. Continue frying while adding half a cup of water and cook until the mixture becomes dry.

In another pan, add oil and fry the whole chicken till golden brown. Allow the chicken to cool. Stuff the chicken with the stuffing mixture along with two boiled eggs. Sew or tie the loose ends of the chicken so that the stuffing does not fall out.

Take a pan, add two to three tablespoons of oil and fry the remaining onions. Add the rest of the ginger-garlic paste, turmeric powder, salt, pepper powder, sauces, vinegar and one cup of water. When the mixture boils, lower the heat and add the chicken, turning it occasionally, and then cover with a lid. Cook until the water dries up and the chicken is done.

Garnish with potato wedges and onions and serve with dinner rolls.

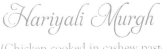

Hariyali Murgh

(Chicken cooked in cashew paste)
(4 TO 6 SERVINGS)

Preparation time	20 minutes
Cooking time	20 minutes

INGREDIENTS

Boneless chicken	500 grams, cut into medium-sized pieces
Garam masala (whole)	1/2 tsp
Onion	1, sliced into small pieces
Turmeric powder	1/2 tsp
Ginger-garlic paste	1 tbsp
Curds	1/2 cup, beaten
Cashew pieces	1/4 cup, ground into a fine paste after roasting
Oil	1/2 cup
Salt	to taste
Green chillies	4 to 5
Fresh coriander leaves	1/2 cup
Mint leaves	10 to 12
Salt	1/4 tsp

METHOD

Grind to paste green chillies, coriander leaves, mint leaves and salt.

Heat oil in a pan and fry the onions till golden brown. Lower the heat and add garam masala, ginger-garlic paste and fry for two to three minutes. Lower the heat and add the chicken pieces. Fry for another two or three minutes. Now add turmeric powder and ground chilli paste and fry till the pungent smell of the raw chilli from the mixture diminishes. Add curd and cook till the oil floats on top. Add one or two cups of water and cook till the chicken is done. Then mix the cashew paste and fry till the gravy thickens and the oil floats on top.

Serve hot with rice or chapatis.

Keema aur Kidney ka Salan

(Minced lamb meat kidney curry)
(4 TO 6 SERVINGS)

Preparation time	10 minutes
Cooking time	20 minutes

INGREDIENTS

Lamb keema	500 grams
Kidneys (lamb)	250 grams, cut into halves
Onion	1, finely chopped
Ginger-garlic paste	1 tbsp
Garam masala powder	1 tsp
Chilli powder	1 tsp
Turmeric powder	1/4 tsp
Curd	1/2 cup
Oil	1/2 cup
Fresh coriander leaves	1/2 cup
Salt	to taste

METHOD

Heat oil in a pan and fry the onions till golden brown. Lower the heat and add ginger-garlic paste, chilli powder, turmeric powder, garam masala powder and salt. Fry while adding a little water. Add the keema and the kidneys and fry until the water from keema dries. Then add the beaten curd and half of the coriander. Cook till the oil floats on top.

Garnish with coriander leaves and serve hot with chapatis.

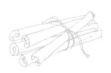

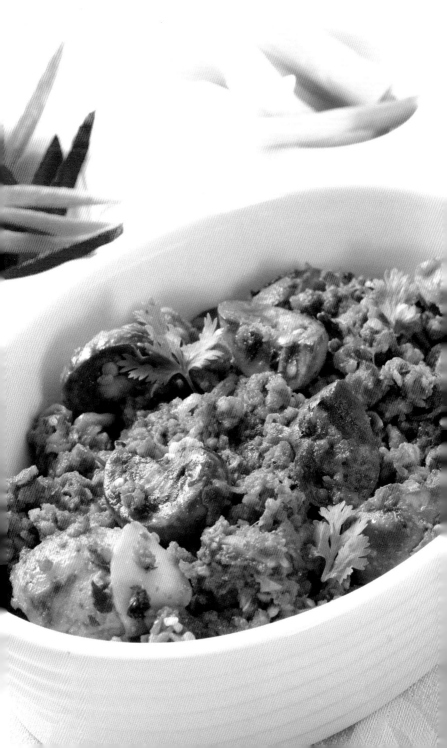

Kacchi Kairee ka Dopiaza

(Mutton cooked with raw mangoes)
(4 TO 6 SERVINGS)

Mutton cooked along with onions and finely-grated raw mango absorbs the subtle flavour of the onions and the tangy flavour of the mango. The tenderizing effect of the ingredients and the thick gravy results in a delightful accompaniment to both rotis and rice.

Preparation time	10 minutes
Cooking time	30 minutes

INGREDIENTS

Mutton with bones	500 grams, cut into medium-sized pieces
Raw mango	1, cut into small pieces
Onion	2, chopped finely
Ginger-garlic paste	1 tbsp
Chilli powder	1 tbsp
Turmeric powder	1/4 tsp
Shah jeera	1 tsp
Oil	1/2 cup
Salt	to taste
Fresh coriander	for garnishing

METHOD

Fry the onions in a pressure cooker with shah jeera till golden brown. Lower the heat and add ginger-garlic paste, chilli powder, turmeric powder, salt and meat pieces. Mix thoroughly and then add two cups of water, pressure cooking till the meat is done. Open the cooker and add the mango pieces, cooking till the oil floats on top.

Garnish with coriander leaves and serve hot with rice or chapatis.

Aloo Badshah ka Korma

(Curry of meat and potatoes cooked with herbs)
(4 TO 6 SERVINGS)

Preparation time	15 minutes
Cooking time	30 minutes

INGREDIENTS

Lamb meat with bones	300 grams, cut into medium-sized pieces
Potatoes	2 to 3, cut into 1-1/2 inch pieces
Onion	1, finely chopped
Ginger-garlic paste	1 tbsp
Chilli powder	1 tsp
Turmeric powder	1/4 tsp
Curd	1/2 cup, beaten
Fresh coriander leaves	1/2 cup
Oil	1/2 cup
Salt	to taste
Khus khus	1 tbsp
Watermelon seeds	2 tbsp
Chirongi	1 tbsp
Shah jeera	1 tsp

METHOD

Dry roast and grind to paste khus khus, watermelon seeds, chirongi and shah jeera.

Heat oil in a pressure cooker and fry the onions with shah jeera till golden brown. Lower the heat and then add ginger-garlic paste, chilli powder, turmeric powder and salt. Stir and add a little water. Add the ground paste and then add the meat pieces, stirring continuously till the oil floats on top. Then add potatoes, half of the coriander leaves and two cups of water. Pressure cook till the meat is done. In case there is water left, cook further.

Garnish with the remaining coriander leaves and serve hot with rice or chapatis.

Safed Machli ka Salan

(Fish cooked in green chillies)
(4 TO 6 SERVINGS)

Preparation time	30 minutes
Cooking time	30 minutes

INGREDIENTS

Fish (fresh water)	1 kg, deboned and cut in 2 inch pieces
Onion	1, finely chopped
Ginger-garlic paste	1 tbsp
Turmeric powder	1/4 tsp
Green chillies	6 to 8, ground into a paste
Hung curd	1/2 cup
Oil	3/4 cup
Salt	to taste
Fresh coriander leaves	1/4 cup, for garnishing
Khus khus	1 tbsp
Watermelon seeds	2 tbsp
Chirongi	1 tbsp
Shah jeera	1 tsp

METHOD

Dry roast and grind to paste khus khus, watermelon seeds, chirongi, and shah jeera.

Sauté fish with oil in a non-stick pan and keep aside.

Heat oil in a pan and fry onions with shah jeera till golden brown. Lower the heat and add ginger-garlic paste, turmeric powder, green chilli paste, salt and the dry roasted paste. Add a little water and fry till the oil floats on top. Now stir in the hung curd and mix thoroughly. Add one cup of water and cook on a slow flame. When three-fourths done, add the fish pieces and cook till the oil floats on top.

Garnish with coriander leaves and serve with rice or chapatis.

Aamchur ke Kofte

(Meatballs cooked with dry mango slices) (Lamb/chicken/turkey)
(4 TO 6 SERVINGS)

Preparation time	30 minutes
Cooking time	20 minutes

INGREDIENTS

Minced meat	300 grams, washed and drained
Onion	1, finely sliced
Ginger-garlic paste	1 tbsp
Chilli powder	1½ tbsp
Turmeric powder	1/4 tsp
Oil	1/2 cup
Dried aamchur slices	10 to 12, soaked in warm water
Dhania powder	1 tbsp
Jeera powder	1 tsp
Coriander leaves	1 tbsp, crushed
Bengal gram	2 tbsp, powdered
Shah jeera	1 tsp
Salt	to taste
Fresh coriander leaves	for garnishing

METHOD

To make the koftas, mix the minced meat, dhania powder, salt, half a tablespoon of chilli powder, shah jeera and the powdered Bengal gram in a bowl. Grind till it forms a thick paste. Make lemon-sized balls out of it and keep aside.

To make the gravy, in another vessel, heat oil and fry the onion till golden brown. Lower the heat and add ginger-garlic paste, the remaining chilli powder, turmeric powder, salt and the crushed coriander leaves. Stir thoroughly till the oil floats on top. Then add the aamchur pieces and four to five cups of water. When the water boils, slowly add the meatballs. Cook till the meatballs are done and the gravy is in a semi-liquid state. If needed, add some more water.

Garnish with coriander and serve hot with rice or chapatis.

Bhagare Ande ka Salan

(Spicy egg curry)
(4 TO 6 SERVINGS)

Preparation time	20 minutes
Cooking time	30 minutes

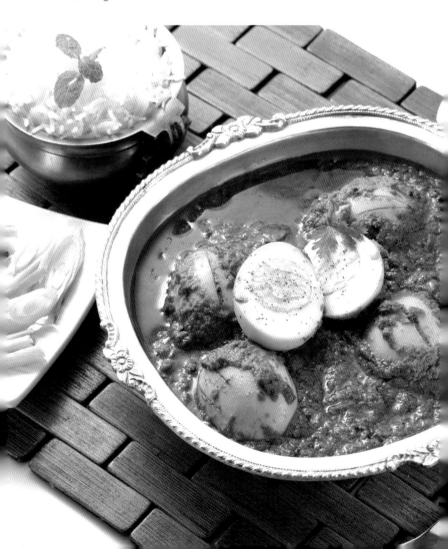

INGREDIENTS

Eggs	6, boiled and peeled
Onion	1, finely sliced
Ginger-garlic paste	1 tbsp
Chilli powder	1 tsp
Turmeric powder	1/4 tsp
Oil	1/2 cup
Tamarind pulp	1/2 cup
Salt	to taste
Peanuts	2 tbsp
Khus khus	1 tbsp
Til (sesame seeds)	1 tbsp
Dry coconut	2 pieces of approximately 2 inches
Dhania	1 tbsp
Jeera	1 tsp

METHOD

Dry roast and grind to paste khus khus, til, dry coconut, dhania and jeera.

Heat oil in a pan and fry the onions till golden brown. Lower the heat and add ginger-garlic paste, red chilli powder, turmeric powder and salt. Add a little water and fry. Now add the ground paste, continue to fry and then add the tamarind pulp. Add half a cup of water while frying. When this is about three-fourths cooked, add the boiled eggs after making a cut on the surface of each egg. Cook till the oil floats on top.

Serve hot with rice.

Aloo ke Dulme

(Stuffed lamb and potato curry)
(4 TO 6 SERVINGS)

Preparation time	20 minutes
Cooking time	30 minutes

INGREDIENTS

Potatoes	6 to 8; peel and scoop in the centre to create a hollow space, deep fry and cool. Also keep aside the scooped portion.
Minced lamb meat	200 grams
Onion	1, finely sliced
Ginger-garlic paste	1 tbsp
Chilli powder	1/2 tsp
Turmeric powder	1/2 tsp
Green chillies	2 to 3, cut into small pieces
Coriander leaves	1 cup, finely chopped
Curd	1 cup, beaten
Oil	1/2 cup
Salt	to taste
Lemon juice	2 tbsp

METHOD

To make the stuffing, wash and cook the minced meat on a slow flame with a little salt, half of the turmeric powder, green chillies, half of the coriander leaves and lemon juice. Cook till the water dries up and the meat is done. Stuff this mixture into the scooped and fried potatoes. Keep aside the remaining keema mixture.

Heat oil in a pan and fry the onions till golden brown. Lower the heat and add ginger-garlic paste, chilli powder, turmeric powder and salt. Fry a little and then add the curd, the remaining minced meat mixture and the scooped portion of the potatoes. Fry for two to three minutes and then add one cup of water. When the mixture thickens, slowly place the stuffed potatoes in it. Cover with a lid and cook on a slow flame till the water evaporates. Stir occasionally and cook till done.

Garnish with fresh coriander leaves and serve hot with rice.

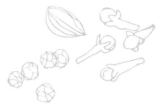

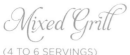

Mixed Grill

(4 TO 6 SERVINGS)

Preparation time	30 minutes
Cooking time	30 minutes

INGREDIENTS

Lamb chops	200 grams, boiled
Kidneys (lamb)	200 grams, cut into 2 halves
Liver (lamb)	200 grams, cut into 2 inch pieces
Tongue (lamb)	2, boiled, peeled and cut into 2 halves
Boneless chicken	200 grams, cut into 5 to 6 pieces
Chicken sausages (optional)	6, cut into 1 inch pieces
Onion	1, finely chopped
Ginger-garlic paste	1 tbsp
Turmeric powder	1/2 tsp
Black pepper	1 tsp
Vinegar	1/2 cup
Soya sauce	1 tbsp
Worcester sauce	1 tbsp
Ajinomoto (optional)	1 tsp
Oil	1/2 cup
Salt	to taste

METHOD

Fry the onions, till golden brown, in a deep vessel. Add the ginger-garlic paste and fry a little. Lower the heat and add turmeric powder, black pepper powder, sauces, vinegar, salt, kidneys, chicken, sausages and the liver pieces. Fry for two to three minutes. Add the stock of the chops or two cups of water and cook till the kidneys are half cooked. Add the chops and tongue and cook till the oil floats on top.

Garnish with potato chips and serve hot with rice.

Muzbi

(Stuffed whole lamb cooked on charcoal)
(10 TO 12 SERVINGS)

The stuffed tender lamb is grilled skilfully and cooked on coal, with blended sauces, to extract varied flavours. This preparation is an art in itself.

Preparation time	60 minutes
Cooking time	90 minutes

INGREDIENTS

Tender lamb (whole)	6 to 8 kgs; with the stomach cleaned, apply ginger-garlic paste and salt all over the meat
Ginger-garlic paste	1 cup
Basmati rice	500 grams, half-cooked
Liver	500 grams
Kidneys	500 grams
Minced meat	250 grams
Tongue	4, boiled and cut into half
Chicken with bones	500 grams
Eggs	6, boiled and peeled
Curd	500 grams
Ginger-garlic paste	2 tbsp
Chilli powder	2 tbsp
Turmeric powder	1 tsp
Shah jeera	1 tbsp
Onion	1, cut into slices
Oil	1 cup
Salt	to taste
Khus khus	2 tbsp
Watermelon seeds	2 tbsp
Fresh coriander leaves	1 cup
Needle and thread	
Charcoal for cooking	

METHOD

Dry roast and grind to paste khus khus, watermelon seeds and coriander leaves.

Heat oil in a vessel and fry the onions and shah jeera till golden brown. Then add ginger-garlic paste, chilli powder, turmeric powder and salt. Stir while adding a little water. Add the ground paste along with the curd, liver, kidneys, chicken, minced meat and cook till the meats are tender and the oil floats on top. Add coriander leaves and mix well. Then add the tongue and eggs.

Take the lamb and stuff this masala and the rice in the stomach. Stitch up the stomach with needle and thread.

Put some oil in a big, flat degh with a lid and place the whole lamb in it. Put the degh on the charcoal. When the lamb gets cooked on one side and becomes brown in colour, turn it over to the other side. Cover the degh with the lid and allow it to cook till it attains a brownish colour on the other side as well. If required, add a little water. The degh should always be covered with the lid when the lamb is being cooked.

Serve with chapatis.

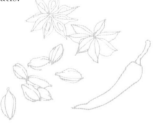

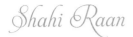

Shahi Raan

(Lamb leg spiced to taste with green chilli paste and yogurt)
(6 SERVINGS)

Preparation time	30 minutes
Cooking time	40 minutes

INGREDIENTS

Lamb leg	1½ kg to 1¾ kg; make deep cuts with a knife on the surface for better marination
Ginger-garlic paste	2 tbsp
Turmeric powder	1/4 tsp
Curd	1/2 cup, beaten
Onion	1, finely cut
Oil	1 cup
Salt	to taste
Khus khus	2 tsp
Chirongi	1 tsp
Watermelon seeds	2 tsp
Cashew pieces	50 grams
Green chillies	10 to 12
Fresh coriander leaves	2 tbsp
Salt	to taste

METHOD

Dry roast and grind to paste khus khus, watermelon seeds, chirongi and cashews. Also grind to paste green chillies, fresh coriander leaves and some salt.

Marinate the leg with salt and ginger-garlic paste for two to three hours. (For best results keep it overnight in a refrigerator.)

In a big kadai, heat oil and fry the whole leg piece on both sides till golden brown. Remove the leg when done and, in the same oil, fry the

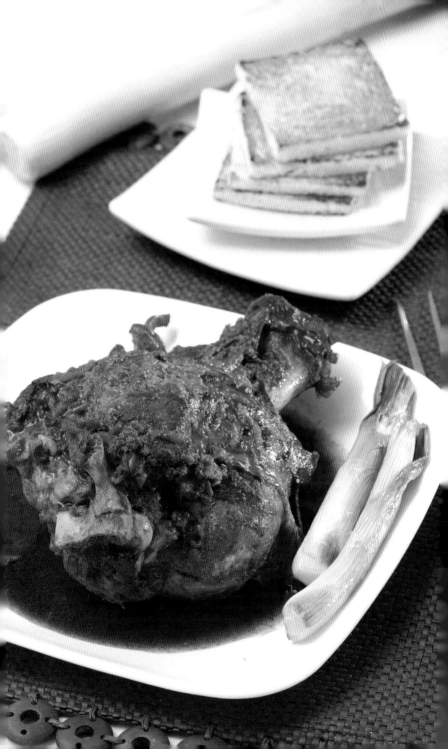

onions with the shah jeera till golden brown. Lower the heat and add the green chilli paste, turmeric powder, dry roast paste and salt. Add some water and fry.

Put the leg piece and the fried masala with three cups of water in a pressure cooker or in a vessel with a lid and cook on low heat till the meat becomes tender.

Garnish with lemon juice and fresh coriander leaves. Serve hot with rice or chapatis.

Paneer Noorjahani

(Cottage cheese in rich, creamy gravy)
(4 TO 6 SERVINGS)

Preparation time	20 minutes
Cooking time	30 minutes

INGREDIENTS

Paneer	200 grams, cut into cubes
Onion	1, cut into thick slices, dry roasted and ground to paste
Cashew	50 grams, dry roasted and ground to paste
Ginger-garlic paste	1 tbsp
Chilli powder	1 tsp
Turmeric powder	1/4 tsp
Oil	1/2 cup
Curd	1/2 cup, beaten
Fresh coriander leaves	1/2 cup
Fresh cream	for garnishing
Salt	to taste

METHOD

Heat oil in a pan, add the onion paste and fry a little. Then add ginger-garlic paste, chilli powder, turmeric powder and salt. Add some water and fry. Then add the curd and fry, then add half of the fresh coriander leaves and a cup of water. When it starts boiling, simmer and add the paneer cubes. Cook till the oil floats on top.

Garnish with cream and fresh coriander leaves. Serve hot with rice or chapatis.

Bharwa Capsicum with Pakodi

(Stuffed capsicum)
(4 TO 6 SERVINGS)

Preparation time	20 minutes
Cooking time	30 minutes

INGREDIENTS

Capsicum	6, cut near the stem and seeds removed
Gram flour	6 tbsp
Chilli powder	1 tsp
Tomato puree	200 gram
Onion	1, finely cut
Chilli powder	1/2 tsp
Turmeric powder	1/2 tsp
Fresh coriander leaves	1/2 cup
Oil	1/2 cup
Green chillies	2, cut into small pieces
Jeera	1 tsp
Lemon juice	2 tbsp
Salt	to taste
Oil	for frying pakodis

METHOD

To make the pakodis, in a bowl, mix the gram flour with a small quantity of chilli powder, salt and water to form a thick paste. Heat oil and fry small quantities of the mixture to form the pakodis. When cool, put the pakodis in a mixer and grind coarsely. To the coarse mixture, add half of the coriander leaves, green chillies and lemon juice. Stuff the capsicum with the pakodi mixture and keep aside.

To make the gravy, fry the onion with jeera in a pan till golden brown. Add turmeric powder, chilli powder and salt. Fry a little, adding a small amount of water. Lower the heat and add the tomato paste and half a cup of water. Stir for two to three minutes and add the stuffed capsicum. Cover with a lid. Cook until the capsicum is a little soft.

Garnish with fresh coriander leaves and serve hot with rice.

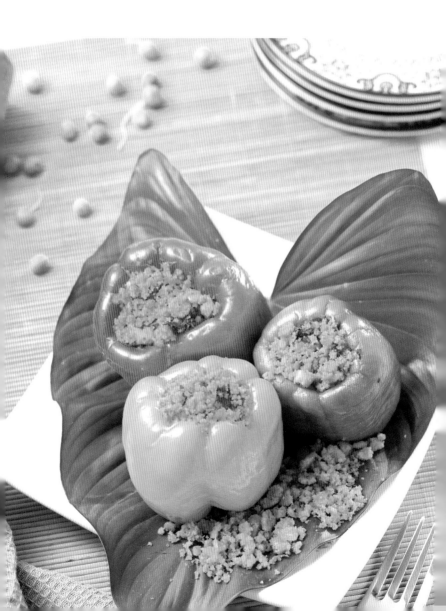

Boondi Methi ki Tarkari

(Boondi cooked with fresh fenugreek leaves)
(6 SERVINGS)

Preparation time	10 minutes
Cooking time	20 minutes

INGREDIENTS

Boondi (made out of gram flour)	150 grams
Onion	1, cut into thin slices
Curd	200 grams, beaten
Ginger-garlic paste	1 tbsp
Chilli powder	1/4 tsp
Turmeric powder	1/2 tsp
Fenugreek leaves	1/2 cup
Oil	1/2 cup
Salt	to taste
Coriander leaves	for garnishing
Lemon juice	for garnishing

METHOD

Heat oil in a pan and fry the onions till golden brown. Lower the heat and add ginger-garlic paste, chilli powder turmeric powder, fenugreek (methi) leaves, salt and a little water. Stir till the oil floats on top. Then add the curd and stir for two to three minutes. Add two cups of water and cook till the mixture reduces to half. Turn off the heat, add boondi and put a lid on the pan.

Garnish with coriander leaves after two to three minutes. Add lemon juice as required. Serve hot with rice.

Gaur ki Phalli aur Besan ke Nimbu ka Salan

(Curry of cluster beans and gram flour balls)
(4 TO 6 SERVINGS)

Preparation time	30 minutes
Cooking time	30 minutes

INGREDIENTS

Gaur ki phalli	250 grams, cut into 1/2 inch pieces
Raw mango	1, cut into pieces
Or dried aamchur pieces	4 to 5, soaked in water
Ginger-garlic paste	1 tbsp
Chilli powder	1 tbsp
Turmeric powder	1/4 tsp
Onion	1, finely chopped
Oil	1/2 cup
Salt	to taste

FOR BESAN KE NIMBU

Besan (gram flour)	150 grams, dry roasted
Chilli powder	1/2 tsp
Turmeric powder	1/4 tsp
Lemon juice	1 tbsp
Fresh coriander leaves	1 tsp
Green chillies	1 to 2, cut into small pieces
Oil	1 tbsp
Salt	to taste
Water	as required

METHOD

To make besan ke nimbu, mix all the ingredients together and make lemon-sized balls out of the mixture. Deep fry the besan balls and keep aside.

To make the gravy, heat oil in a pan and fry the onions till golden brown. Add ginger-garlic paste, chilli powder, turmeric powder, salt and fry by adding water. Then add the gaur ki phalli, mango or aamchur pieces and cook by adding water till the phalli becomes soft. When it is about three-fourths cooked, add the besan balls and cook till the oil floats on top.

Serve hot with rice or chapatis.

Bhagare Tamatar

(Tomato cooked in bhagare baingan masala)
(4 TO 6 SERVINGS)

Preparation time	30 minutes
Cooking time	30 minutes

INGREDIENTS

Tomato (Bangaluri type)	8 to 10, slit on top at four places
Oil	1/2 cup
Tamarind pulp	1/2 cup
Chilli powder	1 tbsp
Turmeric powder	1/2 tsp
Curry leaves	8 to 10
Green chillies	4 to 5, slit into halves
Jeera, rai	1 tsp
Peanuts	2 tbsp
Til	1 tbsp
Dhania	1 tbsp
Jeera	1 tbsp
Dry coconut	4 to 5 pieces of approx. 2 inches each
Salt	to taste

METHOD

Dry roast and grind to paste peanuts, til, dhania, jeera, dry coconut and some salt.

Heat oil in a pan and add jeera, rai and curry leaves to it. When they crackle, lower the heat. Now add the ground paste along with chilli powder, turmeric powder and salt. Stir, adding water till the oil floats on top. Add the tamarind pulp, stir and then add half a cup of water, mixing thoroughly. Add the green chillies and cook till the mixture is about three-fourths cooked. Add the tomato whole. Cover with a lid and cook till the oil floats on top.

Serve hot with rice or chapatis.

Safed Mirchi ka Salan

(Green chilli curry)
(4 TO 6 SERVINGS)

This milk-flavoured side dish made of whole green chillies marinated in lemon juice and cooked in coconut powder makes for a suitable accompaniment to mutton biryani.

Preparation time	15 minutes
Cooking time	15 minutes

INGREDIENTS

Bhajji mirchi	500 grams, deseeded and fried
Jeera	1 tbsp
Lemon juice	4 tbsp
Oil	1/2 cup
Salt	to taste
Til	100 grams, roasted
Dry coconut powder	200 grams

METHOD

Grind to paste til and the dry coconut powder. Heat oil in a pan. Add jeera and when it crackles, lower the heat. Put in the ground paste and salt. Stir while adding water till the oil floats on top. Then add fried chillies, stirring occasionally. Finish with lemon juice.

Serve with chapatis.

Soya Haleem

(Vegetarian haleem)
(4 TO 6 SERVINGS)

Preparation time	15 minutes
Cooking time	60 minutes

INGREDIENTS

Wheat rawa (broken)	250 grams, soaked overnight
Soya granules	250 grams, soaked overnight
Ginger-garlic paste	1 tbsp
Onion	1 tbsp
Red chilli powder	1 tbsp
Turmeric powder	1/2 tsp
Curd	1/2 cup
Garam masala powder	1 tsp
Pure ghee	1/2 cup
Oil	2 Tbsp
Salt	to taste
Fresh coriander and mint leaves	1/2 cup

FOR GARNISHING

Fried onions
Fresh coriander leaves
Lemon wedges
Fried cashew pieces
Pure ghee

METHOD

Cook the soaked wheat rawa in a pressure cooker with water and keep aside. After cooling, grind into paste.

Heat oil in a pan and fry the onion till golden brown. Remove half and keep aside for garnishing. Lower the heat and add ginger-garlic paste, chilli powder, turmeric powder and salt. Drain the soaked soya granules and add to the masalas. Fry till the water evaporates. Then add curd and cook a little.

Take another heavy-bottomed pan. Add the rawa paste, cooked soya curry, ghee, garam masala powder, some fresh coriander leaves and mint leaves and mix thoroughly. If the mixture is thick, then add more water. Place the pan on a low flame and cook the mixture of soya, stirring continuously till the mixture becomes sticky.

Serve hot after garnishing.

Moongodi aur Tamatar ka Salan

(Moongodi and tomato curry)
(4 TO 6 SERVINGS)

Preparation time	15 minutes
Cooking time	20 minutes

INGREDIENTS

Tomatoes	500 grams, cut into small pieces
Moong dal moongodi	150 grams, deep fried till light brown
Onion	1, finely sliced
Ginger-garlic paste	1 tbsp
Chilli powder	1/2 tsp
Turmeric powder	1/2 tsp
Fresh coriander leaves	1/2 cup
Oil	1/2 cup
Salt	to taste

METHOD

Heat oil in a pan and fry the onions till golden brown. Add ginger-garlic paste and lower heat. Add chilli powder, turmeric, salt and half of the coriander leaves and stir for two to three minutes, adding a little water. Add the tomatoes. Cover with a lid and stir occasionally. When half cooked, add the fried moongodis. Cook until the oil floats on top.

Garnish with fresh coriander leaves and serve hot with rice.

Note: Dry soya nuggets can be used as a substitute if moongodis are not available.

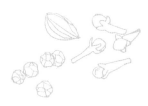

Kulfe ki Bhaji and Chana Dal Curry

(Meat curry with kulfa leaves)
(4 TO 6 SERVINGS)

Preparation time	15 minutes
Cooking time	30 minutes

INGREDIENTS

Kulfe ki bhaji	500 grams or 4 to 5 bunches, washed and cut into small pieces
Chana dal	1 cup, soaked for 1 hour
Tomato	1, cut into small pieces
Onion	1, finely cut
Ginger-garlic paste	1 tbsp
Chilli powder	1/2 tbsp
Turmeric powder	1/2 tsp
Oil	1/2 cup
Green chillies	2 to 3, slit into halves
Curry leaves	4 to 6
Jeera, rai	1 tsp
Raw mango or dry mango	6 to 8 pieces, soaked in water
Salt	to taste

METHOD

Heat oil in a pan. Add the jeera, rai and curry leaves and when they crackle, add the onions and fry till golden brown. Lower the heat and add ginger-garlic paste, turmeric powder, chilli powder, salt, tomato, the bhaji, chana dal, green chillies and the mango pieces. Mix well, adding two cups of water, and cook till the dal is done. If required, add some more water. Cook until the mixture becomes thick and the oil floats on top.

Serve hot with rice.

Bharwa Parval

(Stuffed parval)
(4 TO 6 SERVINGS)

Preparation time	15 minutes
Cooking time	30 minutes

INGREDIENTS

Parval	250 grams, with ends cut and slit 3/4th way into 4 quarters. (Do not cut into 4 pieces; keep one end uncut.)
Jeera powder	1 tbsp
Dhania powder	1 tbsp
Aamchur powder	1 tbsp
Chilli powder	1/2 tsp
Turmeric powder	1/4 tsp
Oil	1/2 cup
Salt	to taste

METHOD

Mix all the dry ingredients together and stuff the mixture into the slit parval. Heat oil in a pan and, on a low flame, put in the stuffed parval and cover with a lid. Cook for approximately fifteen to twenty minutes, stirring occasionally, and then add the remaining mixed masala into the pan. Continue stirring occasionally and cook for another five minutes on low heat.

Serve hot with chapatis.

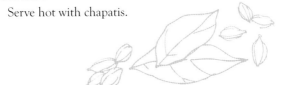

Chukke ki Bhaji aur Pyaz ke Ghatte ka Salan

(Curry of pearl onion in chukke ki bhaji)
(4 TO 6 SERVINGS)

Preparation time	15 minutes
Cooking time	15 minutes

INGREDIENTS

Chukke ki bhaji	500 grams or 5 to 6 bunches, washed and cut into small pieces
Pearl onions	250 grams, peeled
Onion	2, sliced finely
Tomato	1, cut into small pieces
Ginger-garlic paste	1 tbsp
Chilli powder	1 tsp
Turmeric powder	1/2 tsp
Oil	1/2 cup
Salt	to taste

METHOD

Heat oil in a pan and fry the sliced onions till golden brown. Add the ginger-garlic paste, lower the heat and then add the chilli powder, turmeric powder, salt, pearl onions and cook for another minute or two. Add the tomatoes and bhaji and cover with a lid. Stir for two to three minutes. Add a cup of water and cook till the pearl onions are done and the oil floats on top.

Serve hot with rice.

Tomato Moonge ki Phalli ka Salan

(Tomato drumstick curry)

(4 TO 6 SERVINGS)

Preparation time	10 minutes
Cooking time	15 minutes

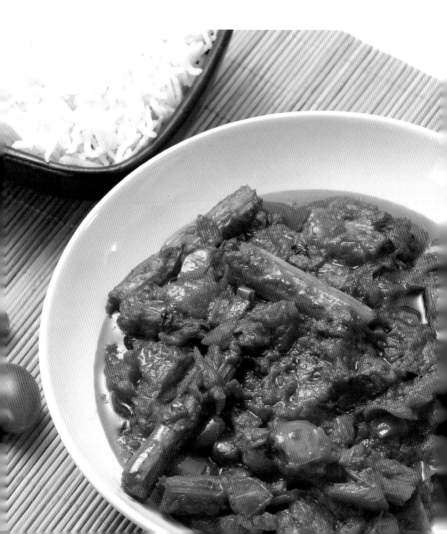

INGREDIENTS

Drumsticks	2 to 3, cut into 2 inch pieces, fried and kept aside
Tomato	4 to 5, pureed
Onion	1, finely sliced
Ginger	1 inch, cut into thin strips
Jeera	1/2 tsp
Chilli powder	1/2 tsp
Turmeric powder	1/2 tsp
Oil	1/2 cup
Salt	to taste
Coriander leaves	for garnishing

METHOD

Fry the onions and jeera in a pan. When the onions become translucent, add the ginger pieces. Fry a little and then add the chilli powder, turmeric powder and salt. Lower the heat and add the tomato puree. Cook till the puree is no longer liquid. Add the fried drumsticks and cook till the oil floats on top.

Garnish with fresh coriander leaves and serve hot with rice or chapatis.

Paneer-Kofte ka Salan

(Paneer kofta curry)
(6 SERVINGS)

Preparation time	20 minutes
Cooking time	20 minutes

INGREDIENTS

Paneer	250 grams
Onion	1, cut into small pieces
Tomato puree	200 ml
Cornflour	1 tbsp
Chilli powder	1/2 tsp
Ginger-garlic paste	1 tbsp
Turmeric powder	1/2 tsp
Jeera powder	1/2 tsp
Oil	1/2 cup
Oil	for frying koftas
Salt	to taste
Fresh coriander leaves	for garnishing

METHOD

To make the koftas, mash the paneer and add cornflour, a small quantity of coriander leaves and salt. Mix well and make lemon-sized balls out of it. Deep fry to golden brown and keep aside.

To make the gravy, heat two to three tablespoons of oil in a pan, add onions and fry till golden brown. Add ginger-garlic paste and fry, adding a little water. Lower the heat and add chilli powder, turmeric powder and salt. Stir and add tomato puree along with a cup of water. Cook until the gravy thickens.

Add jeera powder and the koftas. Turn off the flame and put a lid on the pan after garnishing with coriander leaves.

Serve hot with rice or chapatis.

Rice

Rice is perhaps the most widely consumed staple in India. But rice cooked in the Nizams' kitchens is as different from the everyday boiled or steamed rice made across the country as chalk is from cheese. Long, scented grains are cooked in the dum style—wherein the rice is matured in the gravy or spice mix to fully bring out the flavour and the taste—with mutton, chicken or a combination of vegetables.

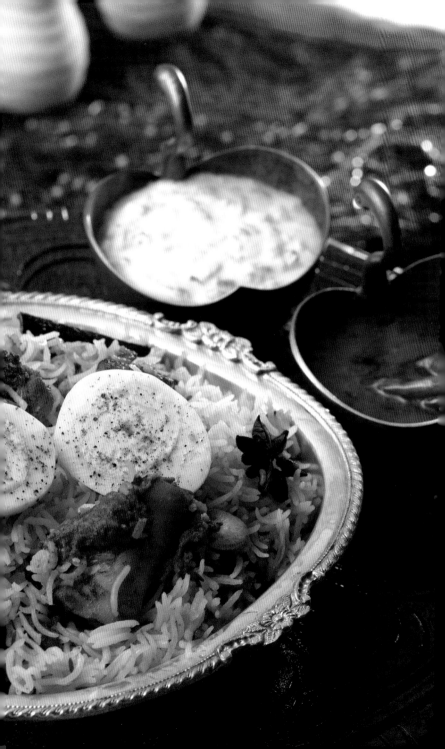

Biryani Golkonda (Kacche Gosht ki Biryani)

(Meat pulao)
(8 TO 10 SERVINGS)

This signature item of Mughlai cuisine is renowned the world over for its subtle flavours and exotic taste. Traditionally, biryani is prepared on a slow charcoal fire (dum). The slow cooking makes the meat tender and succulent, while it absorbs the flavours of the ingredients.

Preparation time	30 minutes
Cooking time	40 minutes

INGREDIENTS

Lamb meat with bones	1 kg, cut into medium-sized pieces
Basmati rice	1 kg
Garam masala powder	1 tsp
Onion	3, finely cut; fry half and keep aside.
Curd	250 grams, beaten
Ginger-garlic paste	2 tbsp
Chilli powder	1 tsp
Turmeric powder	1/2 tsp
Elaichi powder	1 tsp
Garam masala (whole)	1 tsp
Oil	1/2 cup
Pure ghee	1/2 cup
Fresh coriander leaves	1/2 cup
Mint leaves	1/2 cup
Green chillies	4 to 6, cut into small pieces
Saffron	8 to 10 strands, soaked in 2 tbsp of warm milk
Lemon juice	1/4 cup
Salt	to taste

METHOD

In a thick-bottomed pan, fry the remaining onions till golden brown. Add ginger-garlic paste, garam masala powder, elaichi powder and the meat pieces. Fry for two minutes. Add the curd and fry for another couple of minutes. Then add two to three cups of water and cook till the meat is done.

In another pan, heat ten cups of water. Add the whole garam masala and two tablespoons of salt. When the water boils, add the washed rice and cook till the rice is about three-fourths done. Drain the water and remove the rice from the pan.

In a deep, heavy-bottomed pan, layer the pulao by first adding half of the ghee and, over it, half of the rice. Add a layer of the entire cooked meat masala, half of the coriander leaves and mint leaves, half of the fried onions and half of the lemon juice. Layer with the remaining rice, coriander, mint, fried onions, ghee and saffron. Cover the pan with a thin muslin cloth or aluminium foil and then cover with a lid. Cook on medium heat for five to seven minutes, or till the steam comes out. Lower the heat and continue to cook for another seven to ten minutes.

Garnish with fried onions and serve hot with raita.

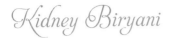 Kidney Biryani

(Kidney pulao)
(4 TO 6 SERVINGS)

Preparation time	20 minutes
Cooking time	30 minutes

INGREDIENTS

Kidneys (goat)	500 grams, cut into halves
Basmati rice	500 grams
Onion	1, sliced
Ginger-garlic paste	2 tbsp
Chilli powder	1 tsp
Green chillies	3 to 4, cut into pieces
Turmeric powder	1/2 tsp
Fresh coriander	1/2 cup
Mint leaves	1/2 cup
Oil	1/2 cup
Pure ghee	4 tbsp
Garam masala powder	1 tsp
Garam masala (whole)	1 tsp
Lemon juice	2 tbsp
Curd	1/2 cup, beaten
Saffron	a few strands, soaked in 1/2 cup of warm milk
Saffron colour (optional)	a pinch, dissolved in 2 tbsp of water
Salt	to taste

METHOD

Heat oil in a pan and fry the onions till golden brown. Remove half and keep aside.

Lower the heat and add ginger-garlic paste, chilli powder, turmeric powder, salt, garam masala powder and the kidneys. Fry, adding a little water, and then add the curd. Stir till the kidneys are cooked. Add more water if required.

Cook rice in a vessel, adding salt and whole garam masala, till it is about three-fourths done. Strain the rice and keep aside.

To assemble, in a thick-bottomed vessel, put two tablespoons of ghee at the bottom and spread half of the rice over it. On this, spread the kidney mixture uniformly and then add the remaining rice over it. On top of the second layer of rice, spread the fried onions, coriander, lemon juice, saffron, colour and the ghee. Cover the vessel with foil and cook on a slow flame for about seven to ten minutes.

Serve hot with raita.

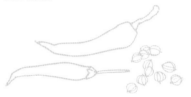

Jhinge ki Biryani

(Prawn pulao)
(6 SERVINGS)

Preparation time	30 minutes
Cooking time	30 minutes

INGREDIENTS

Prawns	1 kg, peeled and deveined
Basmati rice	500 grams
Onion	1, finely sliced
Ginger-garlic paste	1 tbsp
Chilli powder	1 tsp
Turmeric powder	1/4 tsp
Fresh coriander leaves	1/2 cup
Mint leaves	1/4 cup
Garam masala powder	1 tsp
Garam masala (whole)	1 tbsp
Green chillies	4 to 5, cut into small pieces
Lemon juice	2 tbsp
Saffron	a few strands, soaked in 1/2 cup of warm milk
Saffron colour (optional)	a pinch, dissolved in 2 tbsp of water
Ghee	4 tbsp
Salt	to taste

METHOD

Heat oil in a pan and fry the onions till golden brown. Remove half and keep aside.

Lower the heat and add ginger-garlic paste, chilli powder, turmeric powder and salt. Stir while adding a little water. Then add the prawns, garam masala powder, half of the coriander, green chillies and cook till the oil floats on top. Then add lemon juice.

Boil the rice in another vessel, with whole garam masala and one tablespoon of salt, till it is three-fourths done. Drain and keep aside.

To assemble, in a thick-bottomed vessel, put two tablespoons of ghee at the bottom and spread half of the rice over it. On this, spread the prawn mixture uniformly and then add the remaining rice over it. On top of the second layer of rice, spread the fried onions, coriander, lemon juice, saffron, colour and the ghee. Cover the vessel with a foil and cook on a slow flame for about seven to ten minutes.

Serve hot with raita.

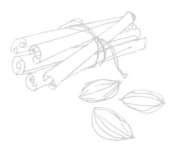

Ande ki Biryani

(Egg biryani)
(4 TO 6 SERVINGS)

Preparation time	30 minutes
Cooking time	30 minutes

INGREDIENTS

Eggs	6, boiled and peeled
Onion	1, thinly sliced
Ginger-garlic paste	1 tbsp
Chilli powder	1 tsp
Turmeric powder	1/4 tsp
Curd	1/2 cup, beaten
Basmati	500 grams
Garam masala powder	1 tsp
Garam masala (whole)	1 tbsp
Lemon juice	2 tbsp
Fresh coriander	1/2 cup
Mint leaves	1/4 cup
Saffron	a few strands, soaked in 1/2 cup of warm milk
Saffron colour (optional)	a pinch, dissolved in 2 tbsp of water
Oil	1/2 cup
Pure ghee	2 tbsp
Salt	to taste

METHOD

Heat oil in a pan and fry the onions till golden brown. Remove half and keep aside.

Lower the heat and then add ginger-garlic paste, chilli powder, turmeric powder and salt. Fry, adding a little water, and then add the curd and half of the coriander leaves and cook till the oil floats on top. Then add garam masala powder, along with the boiled eggs (cut on the top of the surface) and keep the mixture aside.

Cook the rice, with one tablespoon of salt and whole garam masala, till it is about three-fourths done. Strain the rice and keep aside.

To assemble, in a thick-bottomed vessel, put two tablespoons of ghee at the bottom and spread half of the rice over it. On this, spread the egg mixture uniformly and then add the remaining rice over it. On top of the second layer of rice, spread the fried onions, coriander, lemon juice, saffron, colour and the ghee. Cover the vessel with foil and cook on a slow flame for about seven to ten minutes.

Serve hot with raita.

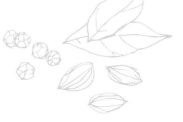

Sabz Nizami Pulao

(Vegetables and rice cooked with spices in Hyderabadi style)
(6 SERVINGS)

Preparation time	30 minutes
Cooking time	30 minutes

INGREDIENTS

Basmati rice	500 grams
Beans	100 grams, cut into 1 inch pieces
Carrot	100 grams, cut into 1 inch pieces
Potato	1, cut into 1 inch cubes
Cauliflower	5 to 6 florets
Peas	100 grams
Tomato	1, cut into small pieces
Curd	1/2 cup, beaten
Onion	1, thinly sliced
Fresh coriander leaves	1/2 cup, finely chopped
Mint leaves	1 tbsp
Oil	1/2 cup
Garam masala powder	1 tsp
Garam masala (whole)	1 tbsp
Ginger-garlic paste	1 tbsp
Chilli powder	1 tsp
Turmeric powder	1/2 tsp
Lemon juice	2 to 3 tbsp
Pure ghee	4 tbsp
Salt	to taste

METHOD

Heat oil in a pan and fry the onions till golden brown. Remove half and
keep aside.

Lower the heat and add ginger-garlic paste, chilli powder, turmeric
powder, salt and all the cut vegetables. Stir till the vegetables are cooked.
Add garam masala powder, green chillies, half of the coriander leaves
and cook till the oil floats on top. Then add lemon juice.

Boil rice in another vessel with the whole garam masala and one tablespoon of salt. Strain the rice and keep aside.

To assemble, in a thick-bottomed vessel, put two tablespoons of ghee at the bottom and spread half of the rice over it. On this, spread the vegetable mixture uniformly and then add the remaining rice over it. On top of the second layer of rice, spread the fried onions, coriander, lemon juice, saffron, colour and the ghee. Cover the vessel with foil and cook on a slow flame for about seven to ten minutes.

Serve hot with raita.

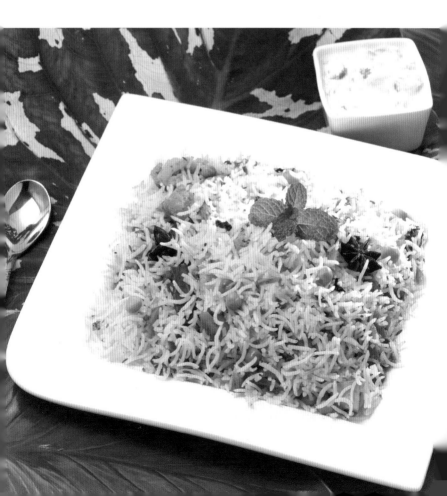

Soya Nuggets ki Biryani

(Soya granules pulao)
(6 SERVINGS)

Preparation time	20 minutes
Cooking time	30 minutes

INGREDIENTS

Soya granules	250 grams, soaked in water for 1/2 hour
Basmati rice	500 grams
Onion	1, thinly sliced
Ginger-garlic paste	1 tbsp
Chilli powder	1 tsp
Turmeric powder	1/2 tsp
Garam masala powder	1 tsp
Garam masala (whole)	1 tbsp
Elaichi powder	1 tsp
Lemon juice	4 tbsp
Saffron	a few strands, soaked in 1/2 cup of warm milk
Saffron colour (optional)	a pinch, dissolved in 2 tbsp of water
Pure ghee	4 tbsp
Oil	1/2 cup
Curd	1/2 cup, beaten
Coriander and mint leaves	1 cup
Green chillies	4 to 5, cut into small pieces
Salt	to taste

METHOD

Heat oil in a pan and fry the onions till golden brown. Remove half and keep aside.

Lower the heat and add ginger-garlic paste, chilli powder, turmeric powder, garam masala powder, salt, elaichi powder and curd. Fry and then add the drained soya granules, half of the coriander, mint leaves and green chillies. Cook till the granules are soft. If necessary, add a little water. Add the lemon juice and keep aside.

Cook rice in another vessel, with one tablespoon of salt and the whole garam masala, till it is about three-fourths done. Drain and keep aside.

To assemble, in a thick-bottomed vessel, put two tablespoons of ghee at the bottom and spread half of the rice over it. On this, spread the curry uniformly and then add the remaining rice over it. On top of the second layer of rice, spread the fried onions, coriander, lemon juice, saffron, colour and the ghee. Cover the vessel with foil and cook on a slow flame for about seven to ten minutes.

Serve hot with raita.

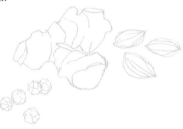

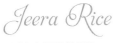

Jeera Rice

(4 TO 6 SERVINGS)

Preparation time	10 minutes
Cooking time	30 minutes

INGREDIENTS

Rice	2 cup
Jeera	2 tbsp
Garam masala (whole)	1/2 tbsp
Ghee	2 tbsp
Green chillies	4 to 5, slit into halves
Fried cashews	for garnishing
Salt	to taste

METHOD

Wash the rice in water and drain. In a heavy-bottomed pan, heat the ghee and add the jeera, garam masala, green chillies and salt. Reduce the heat so that the spices do not burn. Add the washed rice and stir for a couple of minutes. Add four cups of water. When the water boils, lower the heat and cover the vessel with a lid till the water evaporates and the rice is cooked.

Garnish with fried cashews and serve hot.

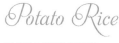

Potato Rice

(4 TO 6 SERVINGS)

Preparation time	20 minutes
Cooking time	20 minutes

INGREDIENTS

Rice	2 cups, cooked
Potatoes	2, cut into small pieces
Onion	1, cut into small pieces
Lemon juice	2 tbsp
Turmeric powder	1/4 tsp
Jeera	1/2 tsp
Curry leaves	4 to 6
Dry red chillies	3 to 4
Fresh coriander leaves	1/4 cup
Oil	2 tbsp
Salt	to taste

METHOD

In a pan, heat oil and add the curry leaves, jeera, dry red chillies, onions and potatoes. Fry till the potatoes become golden brown. Add the turmeric powder, salt, lemon juice and fresh coriander leaves. Mix in the cooked rice and stir for a couple of minutes.

Serve hot with pickle.

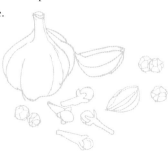

Bhagara Rice
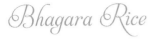

(6 TO 8 SERVINGS)

Preparation time	15 minutes
Cooking time	20 minutes

INGREDIENTS

Basmati rice	500 grams, washed, soaked for 1/2 hour and strained
Dalda ghee	4 tbsp
Garam masala (whole)	1 tbsp
Bay leaves	2
Ginger-garlic paste	1 tbsp
Green chillies	4 to 5, slit into halves
Fresh coriander leaves	1/4 cup
Oil	2 tbsp
Salt	to taste

METHOD

Heat ghee in a vessel and add garam masala. Lower the heat and add ginger-garlic paste, slit green chillies and bay leaves. Fry a little, adding water. Then add the strained rice and salt. Add water in the ratio 1:2 (i.e., one cup rice and two cups of water). When it starts boiling, cover with a lid. Stir occasionally.

When three-fourths of the water has evaporated, cook on a low flame with the lid on till the rice is cooked.

Serve hot with curries or raita.

Dessert

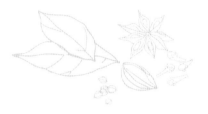

Meetha is possibly the favourite part of any meal for many Indians—
and Hyderabadi desserts will leave them begging for more.
On average heavier than most other sweets of the subcontinent,
these desserts generally contain milk and/or fruit,
and are richly garnished with dry fruits—a very satisfactory conclusion
to your Nizami fine-dining experience!

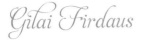

Gilai Firdaus

(Sweet made from pumpkin)
(4 TO 6 SERVINGS)

Preparation time	30 minutes
Cooking time	30 minutes

INGREDIENTS

Pumpkin	1, peeled and grated
Whole milk	2 litres
Sugar	5 tbsp
Elaichi powder	1/2 tsp

FOR GARNISHING

Pineapple pieces and cherries

METHOD

Boil the milk with the grated pumpkin. Stir continuously till it becomes thick. Add sugar and elaichi powder and cool.

Garnish with pineapple pieces and cherries and serve cold.

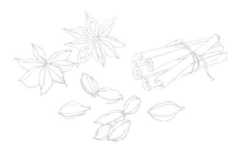

Khubani Trifle
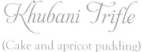

(Cake and apricot pudding)
(4 TO 6 SERVINGS)

Preparation time	30 minutes
Cooking time	20 minutes

INGREDIENTS

Plain sponge cake	200 grams
Apricot	100 grams, soaked overnight, deseeded and cooked with 100 grams of sugar
Milk	1 litre
Custard powder	3 tbsp
Sugar	4 tbsp
Mixed fruit	1 tin, with fruits cut into small pieces
Fanta juice	200 ml
Jam	as required
Dry fruit and fresh cream	for garnishing

METHOD

To make custard, boil milk in a vessel. Add sugar and custard powder mixed with water till the milk becomes fairly thick. Remove and cool.

To assemble, take a bowl that is three inches deep and twelve inches in diameter. Cut the cake horizontally into two halves. Apply jam on both halves. Place both halves together and cut into small squares. Place the cake at the bottom of the dish. Sprinkle Fanta on it so that the pieces are evenly soaked. Now evenly spread the fresh fruits on it. Add the deseeded and boiled apricot with syrup to the layers. Finally, spread the prepared custard. Cool in the refrigerator.

Garnish with cream and dry fruits.

Anokhi Kheer
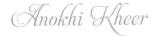

(Pudding with white onion)
(4 SERVINGS)

Preparation time	30 minutes
Cooking time	40 minutes

INGREDIENTS

Whole milk	2 litres
Sugar	4 tbsp
White onion	100 grams, thinly sliced, washed 8 to 10 times in fresh water
Elaichi powder	1/2 tsp
Dry fruits	for garnishing

METHOD

Wash the onion slices thoroughly and boil them till they become soft. Drain the water well.

Boil milk and add the cooked onions, stirring continuously till the mixture becomes homogenous and thick. Then add sugar and elaichi powder and cool.

Garnish with dry fruits and serve.

Shahi Tukde

(Bread pudding)
(6 SERVINGS)

Preparation time	20 minutes
Cooking time	20 minutes

INGREDIENTS

Plain bread	400 grams, with sides removed and the slices cut diagonally into two
Sugar	400 grams
Saffron	a few strands, soaked in 1 tbsp of milk
Elaichi powder	1/2 tsp
Rabdi (thick milk preparation)	250 grams
Dry fruits	for garnishing
Dalda ghee	for frying

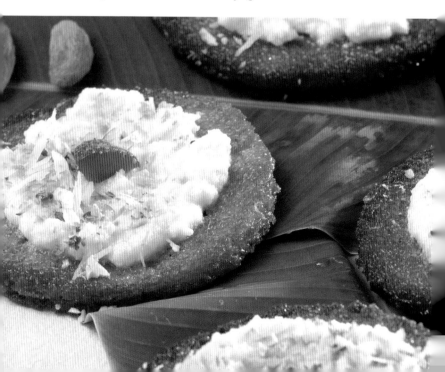

METHOD

Deep fry the bread pieces to golden brown and keep aside.

Melt sugar in a vessel and make a syrup of two-thirds consistency, adding saffron and elaichi powder.

Dip each piece of fried bread into the sugar syrup and arrange them all on a serving plate.

Pour some rabdi on each slice, garnish with dry fruits and serve.

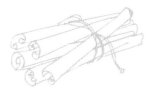

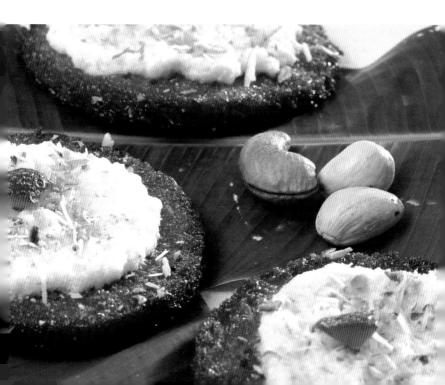

Seetaphal ki Kheer (Seasonal)

(Custard apple pudding)
(4 SERVINGS)

Preparation time	15 minutes
Cooking time	30 minutes

INGREDIENTS

Whole milk	1½ litre
Sugar	4 tbsp
Custard apple	2, deseeded with the pulp retained
Dry fruit	for garnishing

METHOD

Boil the milk in a vessel, stirring continuously, till it gets reduced to half. Add sugar and continue to stir till the sugar is homogenously mixed. After it is cooked, keep the vessel in the refrigerator. Then add the custard apple pulp and mix to attain a uniform mixture.

Garnish with dry fruits before serving.

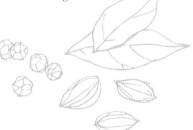

Achaar

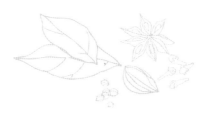

The Hyderabadi pickle is a rare treat for the food lover. Served as an accompaniment with meals, the achaar is meant to provide an added taste of spice. Some of the achaars can be, if stored correctly, preserved for months once prepared. Here I have provided the recipes of four of the signature achaars of the Nizams.

❊

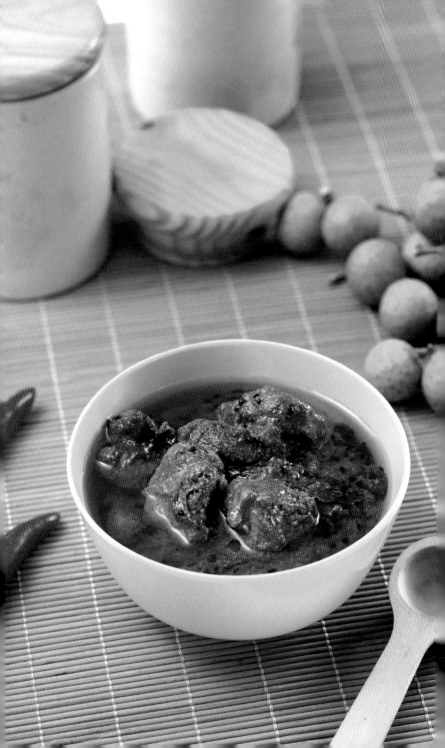

Gosht ka Achaar

(Mutton pickle)

Preparation time	30 minutes
Cooking time	20 minutes

INGREDIENTS

Boneless mutton	500 grams, cut into 2 inch cubes
Chilli powder	4 tbsp
Jeera powder	1 tsp
Rai powder	1 tsp
Vinegar	1/2 cup
Jeera, rai, kalonji	1 tbsp
Oil	1 cup
Salt	to taste

METHOD

Cook the meat by boiling it in two cups of water till it becomes tender and no water remains.

In a pan, pour half of the oil. Heat and add jeera, rai and kalonji, and when they crackle turn off the heat and allow the oil to cool.

In another pan, take the remaining oil and fry the meat pieces. Allow it to cool. Then add chilli powder, rai powder, salt and vinegar. Mix well and then add the oil heated with jeera, rai and kalonji to the meat. Mix and store it in a jar.

If stored in a refrigerator, the pickle can be used for a month.

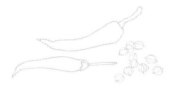

Machli ka Achaar
(Fish pickle)

Preparation time	30 minutes
Cooking time	30 minutes

INGREDIENTS

Fresh river fish	500 grams, deboned and cut into 2 inch cubes
Chilli powder	3 tbsp
Turmeric powder	1/4 tsp
Jeera powder	1 tsp
Lemon juice	1/2 cup
Rai powder	1 tsp
Jeera, rai, kalongi	1 tbsp
Oil	1 cup
Dry red chillies	3 to 4
Salt	to taste

METHOD

Fry the fish pieces in half a cup of oil and keep aside to cool. Heat the remaining oil, add jeera, rai and kalonji, and when it crackles turn off the flame and allow the oil to cool.

Take the fried fish pieces in a bowl and add chilli powder, turmeric powder, salt and lemon juice. Add the cooked tadka (jeera, rai and kalonji) and mix well.

Refrigerate for longer shelf life.

Jhinge ka Achaar

(Prawn pickle)

| Preparation time | 30 minutes |
| Cooking time | 30 minutes |

INGREDIENTS

Fresh prawn	1 kg, washed thoroughly, shelled and deveined
Chilli powder	3 tbsp
Turmeric powder	1/4 tsp
Jeera powder	1 tsp
Garam masala powder	1/2 tsp
Vinegar	1/2 cup
Jeera, rai	1 tsp
Oil	1 cup
Salt	to taste

METHOD

Cook the prawns with salt, turmeric powder and half of the oil till the water evaporates. Allow it to cool.

Take the remaining half of the oil in a pan and heat it. Add jeera and rai, and when the mix crackles, turn off the heat and allow the oil to cool.

Mix the prawns, chilli powder, garam masala powder, salt, vinegar with the jeera-rai oil.

Mix well and refrigerate or store in a cool place.

Aloo-Mirch ka Achaar

(Potato chilli pickle)

Preparation time	30 minutes
Cooking time	30 minutes

INGREDIENTS

Green chillies	100 grams, washed, slit and deseeded
Potato	250 grams, peeled and cut into 1 inch pieces
Mint leaves	1/4 cup
Pearl onion	100 grams, peeled
Garlic	1 pod, peeled
Jeera, rai, kalonji	1 tsp
Vinegar	1/4 cup
Sugar	1 tsp

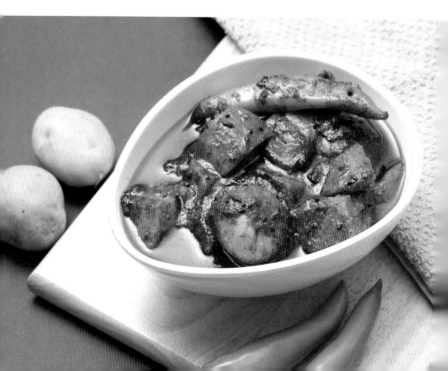

Chilli powder	4 tbsp
Jeera powder	1 tsp
Rai powder	1 tsp
Oil	1 cup
Salt	to taste

METHOD

Heat the oil in a kadai and fry the green chillies till light brown. Remove and keep aside. Fry the potatoes till golden brown and keep aside in a separate vessel.

In the same oil, add jeera, rai and kalonji. When it crackles, turn off the flame and allow the oil to cool.

In a bowl, mix the fried chilli, fried potatoes, mint leaves, garlic, onions, chilli powder, jeera powder, rai powder, salt and vinegar together. Now add the cooled oil with the jeera, rai and kalonji tadka.

Store in a jar and refrigerate.

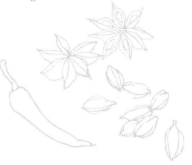

Measurement Table

1 oz	= 28.35 grams	= 1 fl oz	= 30 ml
1 cup	= 210 ml	= 7 fl oz	
1 tsp	= 5 ml	= 1/6 fl oz	
1 tbsp	= 15 ml	= 1/2 fl oz	= 3 tsps

For solids, measure when heaped; for liquids, measure to the brim.

OZ	Grams	OZ	Grams	OZ	Grams	OZ	Grams	OZ	Grams
1/2	15	3	80	5 1/2	155	8	230	10 1/2	305
1	30	3 1/2	95	6	170	8 1/2	245	11	320
1 1/2	40	4	110	6 1/2	185	9	260	11 1/2	335
2	55	4 1/2	125	7	200	9 1/2	275	12	350
2 1/2	65	5	140	7 1/2	215	10	290		

Note: Rounded to multiples of five.

Glossary of Commonly Used Hindi Terms

HINDI	ENGLISH
Arvi	Colocacia
Aamchur	Dry mango
Ambade ki bhaji	Roselle leaves
Aam	Mango
Aloo	Potato
Anardana	Pomegranate
Adrak	Ginger
Badam	Almond
Bandh gobi	Cabbage
Baingan	Eggplant/Brinjal
Besan	Gram flour (Bengal)
Bhindi	Ladyfinger/Okra
Beans ki phalli	French beans
Boot	Green gram
Curry patta	Curry leaves
Capsicum	Bell pepper
Chukandar	Beetroot
Chana	Gram
Chawal	Rice
Cheenee	Sugar

HINDI	ENGLISH
Chigoor	Tender tamarind leaves
Chana dal	Yellow split peas
Chirongi	Piyal seeds
Dahi	Curd/yogurt
Dalchini	Cinnamon
Dal	Lintel
Elaichi	Cardamom
Ghee	Clarified butter
Jeera	Cumin seeds
Jhinga	Prawns
Garam masala	Spice blend
Gehun ka atta	Whole-wheat flour
Gajar	Carrot
Haldi	Turmeric powder
Hara pudina	Mint leaves
Hari mirch	Green chilli
Hara dhania	Coriander leaves
Heeng	Asafoetida
Imli	Tamarind
Kaju	Cashew
Khurbani	Apricot
Kali mirch	Black pepper
Karela	Bitter gourd
Kheera	Cucumber
Khajur	Dates
Khoya	Milk solidified by cooking
Kaleji	Liver
Kesar	Saffron

HINDI	ENGLISH
Kishmish	Raisins
Kadu	Pumpkin
Khus khus	Poppy seeds
Kabuli chana	White gram
Lal mirch	Red chilli
Lauki	Gourd
Laung	Cloves
Lehsoon	Garlic
Moonge ki phalli	Drumsticks
Methi	Fenugreek
Maida	All-purpose flour
Moong phalli oil	Groundnut oil
Moong dal	Yellow split lentil
Matar	Peas
Moongphalli	Peanuts
Namak	Salt
Naariyal	Coconut
Neembu	Lemon
Pakane ka soda	Baking powder
Phool gobi	Cauliflower
Paneer	Cottage cheese
Pyaz	Onion
Pista	Pistachio
Palak	Spinach
Putane ki dal	Bengal gram
Rai	Mustard
Sirka	Vinegar
Sabat kali mirch	Peppercorn

HINDI	ENGLISH
Sonth	Dried ginger
Sooji/rava	Semolina
Saem ki phalli	Val papadi
Tej patta	Bay leaf
Til	Sesame seeds
Turai	Ribbed gourd
Tarbooz seeds	Watermelon seeds
Tava	Hot plate/griddle
Urad dal	Lentil which is white and dried when cooked

Acknowledgements

The success of my first book, *Dastarkhan-e-Moghlai: 101 Easy to Cook Hyderabadi Recipes*, and the number of books sold within India and abroad has infused tremendous confidence in me, enough to undertake writing this book, wherein I have delved into the past to revive some recipes from traditional Mughal cuisine. In my previous book, I had written about dishes that are popular with one and all and easy to cook at home. I have now tried to bring to you delicacies of the past that are relatively unknown and hence have not been experienced by many. This mouth-watering cuisine, with its generous use of spices and careful use of heat, will challenge your senses like no other.

Since the task of compiling these culinary preparations was immense, I thought it fit to seek the help and expertise of my daughters, Anurita, Amrita, Rima and Runa, my sons-in-law, Ravi Kumar, Dr Sanjay Kumar, Dr Anuj Raj and Vishal Karan, all of whom served as tasters for my many experiments.

I would like to thank Shri N. Suresh Reddy, Managing Director, and Shri Akesh Bhatnagar, General Manager, of Golkonda Hotel, Hyderabad, for extending their cooperation in providing photographs for *The Jewels of Nizam*. I would also like to thank Chef Vikas Grover, Golkonda Hotel, for his assistance in the selection of recipes.

I am grateful to my husband, Shri Ashok Kumar, for always supporting me in my efforts and for being a constant source of encouragement and inspiration for my efforts in the culinary arts.

Geeta Devi

About the Author

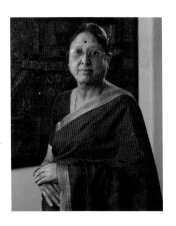

Geeta Devi hails from the Malwala family of Late Raja Dharam Karan of Hyderabad, who came to the city with Nizam-ul-Mulk, the founder of the state.

She has conducted many food festivals in the cities of Mumbai, Kolkata, Chennai and New Delhi, and has received accolades for her knowledge of Hyderabadi cuisine.

She is also the author of the hugely successful *Dastarkhan-e-Moghlai: 101 Easy to Cook Hyderabadi Recipes*.